ttenhouse
1/21/10
$35.00

D0846619

Home Health Care Provider
A Guide to Essential Skills

CUMBERLAND COUNTY COLLEGE LIBRARY
PO BOX 1500
VINELAND, NJ 08362-1500

Emily Prieto, MBA, LSW, started working with the aging population in 1985 as a recreational aide at a day camp for senior citizens in Columbus, Ohio, and was a personal care aide at an Alzheimer's shelter home in Santa Fe, New Mexico. After studying Recreational Gerontology and Sociology, she became a Licensed Social Worker (Ohio) in 1995, working in nursing homes and an adult day care center. Independently, she offered social work consulting to nursing homes in Central Ohio. In addition, she was the Activity Director in an Alzheimer's care facility and an adult day care center, where she also served as the Program Manager. In 2001, she started 2nd Watch Senior Care, a business that provides nonmedical, companion, and errand services to older adults living in the community. She has been a Franklin County (Ohio) Volunteer Guardian for 10 years, serving to direct care and make health care decisions for nursing home residents with limited resources.

Home Health Care Provider
A Guide to Essential Skills

Emily Prieto, MBA, LSW

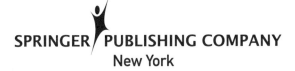

SPRINGER PUBLISHING COMPANY
New York

RA
645.3
P75
2008

Copyright © 2008 Springer Publishing Company, LLC

All rights reserved.

No part of this publication may be reproduced, stored in a retrieval system, or transmitted in any form or by any means, electronic, mechanical, photocopying, recording, or otherwise, without the prior permission of Springer Publishing Company, LLC.

Springer Publishing Company, LLC
11 West 42nd Street
New York, NY 10036
www.springerpub.com

Acquisitions Editor: Sheri W. Sussman
Production Editor: Julia Rosen
Cover design: Mimi Flow
Composition: Apex CoVantage, LLC

08 09 10 11/ 5 4 3 2 1

Library of Congress Cataloging-in-Publication Data

Prieto, Emily.
  Home health care provider : a guide to essential skills / Emily Prieto.
    p. ; cm.
  Includes bibliographical references and index.
  ISBN 978–0–8261–2852–2 (alk. paper)
  1. Home care services. 2. Older people—Care. I. Title.
  [DNLM: 1. Home Care Services. 2. Aged—psychology. 3. Aging.
4. Caregivers. 5. Home Health Aides. WY 115 P949h 2008]

RA645.3.P75 2008
362.14—dc22   2008013306

Printed in the United States of America by Bang Printing.

Contents

Foreword by Todd Gabel, MBA ix

Acknowledgments xi

Introduction xiii

| Chapter 1 | Attitudes of Aging . . . . 1 |

Why This Matters 1
Aging in America: Attitudes on Aging 2
Myths and Facts 3
Normal Aging 5
Summary. 8

| Chapter 2 | Aging at Home. . . . . 11 |

Why This Matters 11
Caregiving and Caregivers 12
Attitudes on Caregiving 13
The Caregiving Community at Home 14
Home Care and Home Health Care 16
The Home Care Industry 21
The Eden Alternative at Home 25
Summary. 27

| Chapter 3 | The Companion Home Care Provider . . . . 31 |

Why This Matters 31
The Companion. 32
Roles and Responsibilities 35
E-mail Correspondence. 36
Emotions of Caring for Others 42
Self-Care 45
Summary. 48

| Chapter 4 | Interpersonal Skills and Communications . . . . 51 |

Why This Matters 51
Personal Skills 52
Communication Skills 52
Communicating With Family. 55

Conversation Skills. 56
Listening Skills. 58
Problem-Solving Skills 60
Conflict-Resolution Skills 63
Decision-Making Skills 65
Observation Skills 66
Summary. 74

Chapter 5   Common Conditions and Diseases of the Aging Body 77

Why This Matters 77
The Aging Body. 78
Alcoholism 79
Alzheimer's Disease 80
Arthritis 84
Bedsores 85
Cancer 86
Congestive Heart Failure (CHF). 88
Constipation 89
Continence. 90
Dementia. 92
Depression 93
Diabetes. 95
Gastroesophageal Reflux Disease (GERD) 96
Hearing Loss. 98
Heart Disease 99
High Blood Pressure (HBP/Hypertension) 100
Impaired and Loss of Vision 102
Kidney Disorder (Renal Disease) 103
Lung Disease 104
Mental Health 106
Osteoporosis. 107
Pain 108
Parkinson's Disease. 109
Stroke (CVA/Cerebral Vascular Accident) 112
Physicians and Specialists 113
Summary. 114

Chapter 6   The Terminally Ill Client 117

Why This Matters 117
A Terminal Diagnosis. 118
Hospice Care. 120
Summary. 122

Chapter 7   Caring for Couples 125

Why This Matters 125
Caring for Couples 126
Situations of Partner Care. 126
Emotions of Partners in Care 126
Defining Couples 128

Respite Care 129
Summary. 129

Chapter 8   About Activities 131

Why This Matters 131
Doing Things. 132
Activities and Quality of Life 132
Activities of Life and Activities of Recreation 135
A Companion's Role in Activity Planning. 137
Be Prepared With Activities. 139
Activity Ideas 140
Summary. 157

Chapter 9   Planning and Preparing Meals 163

Why This Matters 163
Nutrition, Eating, and the Aging Body 164
Involving the Client in Meal Planning and Preparation 169
Shopping for the Client 171
Recipes 173
Summary. 180

Chapter 10   Home Safety and Household Management 183

Why This Matters 183
Keeping the Home Safe. 184
Emergencies. 205
Telephone Contact 207
Household Management 208
Universal Design 210
Summary. 212

Chapter 11   Legal Authority and Money Matters 215

Why This Matters 215
Decision Making and the Older Adult. 216
Legal Tools and Designations for Health Care Decision Making 216
Money Matters: Medicare and Medicaid 220
Summary. 221

Chapter 12   Planning for Placement 223

Why This Matters 223
Facilitating Long-Term-Care Planning 224
Moving From Home 224
Living Options and Alternatives 226
Visiting and Evaluating Health Care Facilities 229
The Companion's Role After Facility Placement. 234
Summary. 235

References. 237

Index 239

Foreword

I am sure that you have been told on numerous occasions, "I could never do your job." It takes a special person to devote a career to caring for seniors. Individuals who devote their lives and livelihood to this profession are often the unsung heroes of our nation's frail senior population. Care providers play many vital roles in the lives of the individuals they work with and the families of their clients. Care providers wear many hats during any given day, such as caretakers, friends, confidants, event planners, chefs, and sounding boards. In a society that places so much value on technology and high speed, the skillful ability to slow down and listen to the thoughts and feelings of an individual are too often overlooked.

As our population continues to age and the adult children of the "Greatest Generation" are pulled in increasingly varied directions, the demand and necessity of formal care providers will continue to increase. I have had the opportunity to work in a variety of states for organizations providing long-term care. Each time I have attended a forum or a discussion group involving family members caring for their loved one at home, the experiences shared by families using home care providers and personal care assistants is always positive and uplifting. Often families considering an assisted living situation will share their heartfelt gratitude toward their extended family member, the formal care provider. Many families rely on the opinion of the formal care provider during the decision-making process of transitioning to an assisted living or skilled nursing facility.

Many families who do decide to transition their loved one from home to a residential setting also elect to retain the services of the care provider. This decision is of great value not only to the care recipient but also to the facility staff and the care recipient's family. The families and the facility benefit from the role of the formal care provider as a liaison between the facility and family. Care recipients benefit from retaining a familiar friend during a time that can be traumatic. The care provider also benefits by expanding their exposure to other families who may wish to hire the individual to provide extra services and companionship to their loved one.

Whatever the services and wherever they are provided, there is no doubt that the role of the formal care provider is vital to our aging population. You have selected an admirable profession and you are taking an important step by seeking additional knowledge about your work. I like to think that what you do shapes who you are and who you are shapes what you do. As you continue to grow in your personal and professional endeavors, perhaps you may wish to consider the words of Mahatma Gandhi as your mantra: "My life is my message."

—Todd Gabel, MBA
Senior Executive Director, Sunrise Senior Living, Columbus, OH
Owner, TFG Consulting, Columbus, OH

Acknowledgments

First, I would like to thank every person over the age of 65 who I have worked with, for sharing their experiences during the aging process. I am indebted to them for the wisdom and vision I gained through their storytelling. I am particularly grateful to the clients and family members of 2nd Watch Senior Care for allowing me into their homes and lives; without their support, this book would not have been possible.

I would like to express my gratitude to Sheri W. Sussman at Springer Publishing Company, who recognized my passion for working with the elderly and maintained confidence in my ability to educate others.

A special thank you to Paul Dravillas, who created the original artwork from which the illustrations were derived. I would like to acknowledge Dean Cox for his graphics and Dennis Trucks for the continuous technical assistance.

For encouraging this opportunity and his support, I thank my husband, Tom.

Introduction

In the dozen years I have worked in geriatrics, I have repeatedly been asked for advice on managing issues of aging, from daily care concerns to long-term-care planning to end-of-life decision making. Questions have come from family caregivers, coworkers, friends, neighbors, and other health professionals. I have been encouraged by numerous people to share my experiences and knowledge because understanding the diverse issues of aging takes time and awareness. This manual has given me the opportunity to organize answers to those questions, provide other information, and to grow personally and professionally.

My experiences as a Geriatric Social Worker and Activity Director in nursing homes and an adult day care center led me to venture into the business of providing home-based, nonmedical support services to the aging. This experience reinforced my recognition of the growing need for community-based care and support for home-care clients. The success of this service has truly been an advocacy for home-care recipients while observing the enhancement of quality in daily life.

As in any profession, industry terminology is used to characterize and communicate a concept while the general public has other meanings and perceptions. Some professionals debate the definitions and distinctions between a caregiver and a caretaker, though the dictionary makes slight differences between the two terms. Merriam-Webster Dictionary (2007–2008) defines a *caregiver* as "a person who provides direct care (as for children, elderly people, or the chronically ill)" while the definition of a *caretaker* is "one that gives physical or emotional care and support." In this manual, the term *caregiver* will be used to refer to family members providing care and the terms *companion* and *home care provider* refer to the formal care providers who are hired to give assistance. The term *companion* implies assistance with Instrumental Activities of Daily Living, not assistance with personal care routines, while home care providers may offer support with either Instrumental Activities of Daily Living or Activities of Daily Living. The information in this book focuses on nonskilled care practices and those who provide nonmedical support services, by a companion or home care provider; therefore, these two terms will be used interchangeably. The terms *care recipient* and *client* are used interchangeably to refer to the person receiving care.

This manual emphasizes the positive interaction between care recipients' psychological and social functioning. The care recipients' ability to connect personal perceptions and behaviors with their home and community environments contributes to healthy aging. The medical approach for treating illness may be necessary; of equal significance to physical health is the enrichment of psychosocial well-being by valuing the components of everyday life.

How to enhance aspects of everyday life is the focus of this book. Methods are offered for improving interpersonal communications that can lead to successful, personal, and professional interactions. Creative recipes are presented to meet special and restricted diets; as well, these user-friendly recipes do not involve extensive ingredients or time. The innovative, one-on-one activity ideas are techniques for building care provider–care recipient relationships. Information on age-related illnesses and diseases (signs, symptoms, and treatments) provides a general base of knowledge necessary for care providers. The chapters "Caring for Couples" and "The Terminally Ill Client" offer perspectives on caring for these unique populations. Companions and care providers new to home care and working with the aging population will learn the basics of quality service delivery, while readers who have experience with the home care industry will glean new ideas to improve care and service.

The unspoken knowledge of giving excellent care comes from genuinely understanding the care recipient. At the end of the day, the quality care provider will have provided ease and comfort to the care recipient, which family members will also witness through the exceptional care given to their loved one. This book is for anyone who strives to provide this level of intimate care.

Beyond the challenges and losses of working with the aging population are the satisfactions, achievements, and unforgettable experiences of life and death that teach the willing learner about adapting to change throughout one's lifetime—the process of aging.

Attitudes of Aging

1

In This Chapter, You Will Learn

1. Perceptions and attitudes about aging

2. Myths and facts related to aging

3. Aspects of normal and successful aging

Why This Matters

Aging is a way of life in all societies. Attitudes about aging influence the way people age and how society responds to their aging population. A general understanding of the physical and psychological characteristics of the aging process will promote sensitivity to the needs of this group; thoughtful attention can change the methods of care and treatment. Aging adults want to be considered as an integral, teaching component of their society. They want to be taken care of with respect and dignity. They want care providers to treat them with compassion. Care providers help individuals through the aging process by allowing them time to talk about their life experiences in a supportive environment where fears and feelings can be expressed safely.

Aging in America: Attitudes on Aging

Aging in American society is viewed as a disease in and of itself. We are conditioned to believe that with age comes dependence and the need for care by doctors, nurses, and aides through hospitalizations, medications, and nursing homes. Some older adults are affected by disease and have to rely on others for assistance or care, though this does not happen to every person over the age of 65. There is an attitude in America that becoming an older adult is undesirable. We are taught that older age is a depressing life stage of disease and dependence. The misperception of aging and being an older adult is that pain and sickness are inevitable and that we will become a burden to our family and society. We are socialized to accept that the aged are not an integral piece of society because there is no personal or social value to being an older adult. Inactivity and lack of productivity does not naturally occur with older age. Older adults continue to contribute to society and their communities. Some people choose to be less active in their older years while others volunteer regularly for charitable organizations, write novels, and win the Nobel Peace Prize. Aging men and women who are able to participate in life activities and seek such opportunities are plentiful. Society is slowly beginning to acknowledge the value in life experiences and teachings that the aging population has to offer, which means that older adults will be listened to with worth and respect.

The fear of aging and becoming an older adult permeates American society. A variety of business industries have developed products and services to meet the demands and expectations of the aging population. These products and services represent a myriad of concerns from aesthetic to serious medical provisions. The cosmetic industry sells face, hair, and body products to manage the perceived negative changes of our physical appearance in age. This reinforces fears of physical (weight gain, supple skin) and aesthetic (wrinkles, gray hair) changes that can naturally occur in age. Media, movies, and magazines portray the aged as pleasantly confused and forgetful grandparents, crotchety neighbors, erratic drivers, and helpless old ladies or men. This perpetuates the fears of a changing physical appearance as well as draws attention to a changing mental status and the inability to act appropriately. Pharmaceuticals largely serve the aging population, particularly through medications, supplies, and equipment. Products' marketing reminds consumers that life will be more comfortable and maybe longer with their use because we are afraid of what life might be like without them. The focus on illness by the insurance industry emphasizes the many afflictions that can occur with age; then, they endorse the use of medications or special treatments to prevent these potential concerns. Additionally, the insurance industry has long-term-care insurance policies, which could reassure a person that costs will be affordable just in case long-term placement is necessary. These policies can be extremely beneficial; even still, it is a planning tool sold on the fear of high health care costs. Banking and financial industries encourage young and old alike to save money through investment opportunities drawing on the fear that financial resources will not be available in later life. Society is fearful of growing old because we are told and taught to be through American culture and commerce.

Consider how elders are treated in other countries and cultures. In the Worldmark Encyclopedia of Cultures and Daily Life, editor Timothy Gall points out that men of Malaysia are honored at the age of 60, considered a "landmark age," with a celebration for longevity and good health (1998, p. 466). In Japan, September 15 is a holiday honoring the elderly (Gall, 1998). Aged persons are cared for by their children and are not placed in care facilities in Libya, a country in North Africa (Gall, 1998). How and why did growing older in the United States become a negative experience when it happens to every one of us?

An aging adult in America does have advantages. Government-sponsored programs of housing and home- or community-based care are available. Medicare, a federally funded program, provides medical insurance to those over 65. Tax benefits and utility-assistance programs exist for those over 65 who meet specific criteria. Some families treat their elders as leaders, considered as matriarchs (female) or patriarchs (male). Members of society who respect aging adults may be inclined to open doors and give up their seat or place in line to an older adult. As there is negative discrimination against the aging, so there is also positive discrimination.

The most unfair attitude toward the aging is ageism, when a person is treated as "old" because of the number of years he or she has lived. Ageism encourages segregation, further isolating older adults from general society. This attitude creates feelings of abandonment and loneliness in older adults. Identifying ageism in the workplace can be a legal challenge, yet people do claim they have been discriminated against because of their age. Families also practice ageism by attempting to overprotect older family members from certain circumstances common to the aging process. However, popular culture tells us that age is an attitude, and that a person is only as old as he or she thinks they are. At 90 years, an individual may function as if he or she was 60 years and may be referred to as active, full of life, and "young-old," which is an older person who may look or act younger than how a person at that age is *expected* to look or act.

The practice of applying negative *or* positive stereotypes can be impractical and destructive, as stereotypes of any type set up society and individuals for a failure of perceived expectations. It goes against the calm, quiet, and serene stereotype when the sweet-looking 90-year-old woman is irritable, argumentative, and demonstrates inappropriate actions even though there may be emotional or physical reasons for her attitude and behaviors. The aging process is as personal and unique as each individual.

Myths and Facts

In addition to stereotypes, there are myths and facts that positively and negatively influence the perception of aging. A commonly believed myth is that age, especially old age, causes sickness and disease. Unhealthy habits may take a physical toll on the body over the years and there are diseases associated with age, though younger people can have cancer, heart disease, diabetes, strokes, and Parkinson's disease. Depression is seen in the aging population though not every older adult suffers from severe depression, the numbers are not overwhelming. The National Institute of Mental Health (2007) reports 2 million (5.7%) out of 35 million Americans over 65 suffer from severe depression and 5 million (14%) experience less severe forms of depression. Depression in older adults is a serious condition that certainly needs further research and attention.

Particularly with the introduction of long-term-care insurance policies, many assume living in a nursing home in later life is inevitable. The Administration on Aging through the U.S. Department of Health and Human Services (2007) reports that only 4.5% of persons 65 and over lived in nursing homes in 2000. This number increases to 18.2% for those over 85 years. A major function of the booming home health care industry is keeping older adults living in their homes longer and, as appropriate, avoiding nursing home placement. See Tip 1.1 for more information about the profiles of aging adults in America.

The perception that older adults lack the ability to make good decisions is yet another myth. Not all older people are dependent on others for decision making and problem solving. Family members and care providers may not agree with decisions made by an older adult, though this does not always mean that those decisions are wrong. Many older adults continue to use their knowledge and experience to adjust to new situations and are willing to learn new skills, which is indispensable for adapting to challenging circumstances.

Tip 1.1

Profile: Statistics of an American Adult Over 65 Years

36.8 million people over 65 in 2005, an increase of 9.4% since 1995
About one person out of eight in the population is an older adult
In 2005, over 2 million people celebrated their 65th birthday
In 2000, the 85+ population was 4.2 million; in 2030, the same population is projected to increase to 8.9 million
In 2005, 18.5% of people 65+ were minorities:

African American 8.3%
Asian or Pacific Islander 3.1%
American Indian or Native Alaskan less than 1%

In 2005, 72% of men were married while 42% of women were married
In 2004, 43% of older women were widows
About 30% (10.6 million) noninstitutionalized older adults live alone: 7.7 million women and 2.9 million men
50% of women over 75 live alone
In 2000, 4.5% (1.56 million) of the 65+ population lived in nursing homes
In 2000, 4.7% of the 75–84 population lived in nursing homes
In 2000, 18.2% of the 85+ population lived in nursing homes

Note: Information retrieved from the U.S. Department of Health and Human Services, Administration on Aging, http://www.aoa.gov/press/fact/pdf/ss_stat_profile.pdf

Some facts of physical and physiological aging do support these myths. Obvious physical changes that occur with age are gray hair and wrinkles. We may notice a large number of older adults wearing glasses, hearing aids, or dentures to compensate for the changes, though not every aging person needs large print or loud volume just because they have lived many years. The skin loses elasticity and becomes drier, appearing dehydrated and in need of moisturizing. Sensory perceptions decrease with age. A change in one or all of the senses of vision, hearing, tasting, and smelling usually occurs. The sensation from touch or tactile stimulation is also subject to diminish. Physiologically, bodily responses slow down. It takes the body longer to receive messages from the brain, such as to move the right foot or left arm, which may be compounded by chronic conditions that are prevalent in the aging body. Changes in elimination processes, eating habits, and sleep patterns are also known to occur with age. Mood or personality changes can be symptomatic of a disease process or the result of inadequate coping methods to manage the current circumstances or the aging body. A person who had been outgoing may become withdrawn and a fun-loving person can become angry in older years. While these age-related changes sometimes occur, not all of them will happen. The advancement of science and technology (including medications) as it relates to aging may alter the process of aging as we know it.

Normal Aging

After considering stereotypes, myths, and facts, is there such a thing as normal aging? What does normal aging look like? Rather than viewing stereotypes, myths, and facts as inevitable changes for all people, they can be seen as scenarios and possibilities that allow one to plan for what could occur through the aging process. Instead of assigning positive and negative values, the aging process should be understood and experienced as what it is: a transformation. Therefore, emotional, physical, and physiological changes *are* normal aging.

The ability to accept and cope with ongoing change is the essence of aging. To age normally is to accept the ups and downs, the advantages and disadvantages, of the aging process. Accepting change is easier said than done and can be complicated by external issues. The physical environment may no longer be suitable and living space often becomes unmanageable. A smaller home may be ideal or home adaptations may be needed for the older adult to function in the home. Disease or chronic conditions may require constant medical supervision necessitating care-facility placement. Relationships with family and friends can become strained both with continuous added demands and when difficult decisions have to be made. The unplanned event of a fall resulting in broken bones, the death of a spouse, or the sudden onset of a disease or condition changes circumstances that impact how normal aging continues.

Think about this: In our formative through young adult years, we are taught to plan for an independent life. We prepare for a productive career through training and education, and work to accomplish personal and professional goals. Throughout this learning process, we become self-sustaining and self-reliant. Our character and values are solidified over the 50 (give or take) years of practice. Personal expectations are fulfilled; social obligations are satisfied. Older age comes and those years of practice and routine require adaptation. There has been no emotional training for the need for assistance or dependency. A stroke that alters mobility now necessitates the use of a cane, walker, or wheelchair. Because the vocabulary has been minimized and the ability to speak restricted, a pad of paper and pen is necessary to communicate. Instead of going to work, 3 hours each morning is now spent getting dressed, eating, and resting. This way of life is unlike how it was previously known.

Older adults are faced with internal emotions regardless of external conditions that can occur. Feelings of neglect, abandonment, and isolation are common, and can become more prevalent after a person has been forced to change their living situation. Some aging people struggle to cope with the changing sense of autonomy and independence. There is often a looming fear of being placed in a nursing home or other type of care facility. Not knowing how life will unfold influences or impedes planning and decision making. Some older adults review unresolved conflicts or past perceived failures that can result in guilt or depression. Grief occurs over the loss of mental or physical health status and at the death of family members and friends. Real or potential health issues are frequent concerns. Abuse is a very real threat for too many older adults, and too often others use manipulation to achieve their desired results.

The idea of dependency is a common preoccupation with aging adults. The independent, aging adult fears that there may come a day when he or she will have to rely on family members, friends, or professionals for assistance with transportation, financial affairs, personal care, and other routine tasks. Asking for help is considered an act of dependence and being dependent on others is not a comfortable concept for most people. Particularly in American society, a number of people perceive minimal dependency and asking for help as a loss of dignity. Over the years of creating an independent, self-sufficient life, some people never learn how to ask for help; for some, asking for help only comes in older age. The reluctance and resistance to ask for assistance when it is needed can lead to feelings of anger, frustration, and even injury while a person tries to manage life matters. The aging adult may have to make great effort not only to accept help from others, but to admit that the help is necessary. Maintaining personal dignity and integrity is at the core of dependency. Is the person who desperately needs help but does not ask for it still maintaining their dignity and integrity? The questions concerning the what and how of dependency are changing to more tolerable definitions of need and support. Is an aging person who needs hired transportation to the grocery store dependent? If so, is the 30-year-old adult who takes a bus or taxi to the grocery also dependent? Is the 75-year-old woman who never managed household finances because her now-deceased husband always did considered dependent because she needs help with paying bills in a timely manner? Is an 80-year-old man thought to be dependent when he hires someone to prepare meals because his wife, with Alzheimer's disease, can no longer do it?

The older adult is likely managing the demands of daily life while coping with these potentially overwhelming thoughts and feelings. Many older adults remain involved in their money matters, not only deciding on how money will be saved or spent for future use but also ensuring that current bills are paid on time. Telephone calls to the bank, financial planner, and utility companies take time. It can be difficult for older adults to physically manipulate the small buttons on telephones or they may be unable to navigate through the automated systems fast enough, which may terminate the call. Daily medication schedules can be demanding. The majority of older adults take responsibility for managing their medications, which can become a time-consuming schedule for those who take multiple medications. Keeping track of when each medication is taken, how it should be taken (with or without food or drink), and if medications will negatively interact with others requires time and effort. Dropping off and picking up prescriptions takes time and transportation, and may require frequent interactions with a doctor or pharmacist to learn medication side effects and effectiveness. A person who has specialized medical treatments, such as dialysis or chemotherapy, has additional considerations. Appointments and schedules are other demands. For older adults who no longer drive, transportation must be coordinated. The older adult may need another person to sit at the appointment to help with understanding information and instruction. There can be long waits at the doctor's office that may interfere with other appointments, activities, and medication schedules, or sitting too long may become physically uncomfortable. Household management and recreational pursuits are yet additional demands, wants, and needs of daily life. A schedule full of finances, medications, and appointments can minimize the attention spent on other aspects of daily life.

Social stimulation can be an important feature of successful aging for those who find satisfaction in being around others. Research indicates that an adequate amount of human interaction adds quality and longevity to life. Many aging adults plan or attend social events because they have enjoyed social interactions throughout life or because they subscribe to the notion that social interactions have therapeutic benefits. Socializing creates learning opportunities through discussions of thoughts and experiences. Talking with others presents occasions for gaining new information, including methods for coping during the aging years. People share past and current achievements and experiences when interacting with others, creating environments that validate the self. For some, socializing may need only to be exposure to others at the grocery store or going to the library once a week; for others, being active in daily or weekly events is necessary for meeting social needs. Socialization is critical for people with physical or mental limitations; whether or not a person is able to express satisfaction, being with individuals or part of a larger group may be their only occasion to feel connected with other humans and not feel alone. Social needs vary for each person. The depth and length of interactions may not be as important as simply having opportunities to socialize with others.

Spiritual or religious beliefs are extremely important to many people throughout the aging process. Spirituality is belief in personal values and something greater than the self that fulfills needs of connectedness to the world and a higher power. Religions (Christianity, Buddhism, Hinduism, Muslim, and Judaism) are specific organized systems of beliefs and behaviors, which also serve to connect individuals to humanity and a greater power. Aging people use their spirituality and religion to guide them through changing life processes to cope with loss and, ultimately, death.

Personal experiences and cultural backgrounds shape spiritual and religious belief, ultimately influencing attitudes of aging and illness. The cause of disease and illness is explained differently from culture to culture or religion to religion. Some Spanish societies believe illness is the result of God's punishment, while cultures of the Caribbean Islands believe evil spirits and demons invade the body. Most European Americans view disease as the result of self-inflicted, negative behaviors. The value systems of personal and cultural customs shape how adults are cared for during the aging process. For example, not every religion or culture accepts the role of a medical doctor for health care intervention. Asian and Hispanic Americans use healers as health care providers, while Native Americans bring shamans, or medicine men. Some African American cultures rely on folk practitioners, who use a blend of herbs, plants, and roots for medicinal cures. Methods of treatment are not always medical; plenty of cultures use diet and home remedies to treat illness while others rely on herbs and plants as medicinal cures. Many cultures and spiritual or religious people use prayer as a means of treatment.

Aging is a natural stage in the process of life for any person, of any culture or religion, in any geographic region of the world. Spirituality, religion, and culture significantly influence how people age and how elders are treated within a society. The societal perception of illness and aging will shape the care and treatment of this population. Every individual is accountable for aging gracefully, which occurs when an aging adult is able to accept the benefits and challenges of older adulthood and the aging process. A person who learns to accept and adapt to changing physical or emotional abilities and possibly social roles can age successfully.

Summary

Social attitudes about aging influence the way people age and how cultures respond to the wants and needs of this population. Business and commerce in the United States is both manipulating how we age and simultaneously creating necessary markets to meet the exclusive needs of the aging population. The banking, cosmetics, pharmaceutical, and housing industries persuade the general public on how to age and what to anticipate from the aging process. Other industries are influenced by the demands of this population, such as the housing industry building easily adaptable living spaces for the aged or disabled.

Myths perpetuate positive and negative attitudes toward aging that can create unfair expectations of how individuals should age and the type of care provided to aging adults. Facts do support some myths about aging, though every person should be treated as an individual through this unique process. Ageism, the prejudice against an older adult because of the number of years they have lived, results in the further isolation of older adults from society.

The aging process is a range of physical, mental, and emotional demands. Adapting to new situations, medical routines, and shifting social roles can become overwhelming while maintaining daily life. Furthermore, many older adults contemplate possible future vulnerabilities, such as disease and dependency. Appropriate socialization can add to quality of life by minimizing feelings of isolation and abandonment. Social and cognitive stimulation contribute to successful aging. Normal aging is the ability to accept and cope with changing emotional, physical, and physiological needs.

Questions

How does society influence the aging process?
Are stereotypes helpful in working with the aging population?
Name two myths about aging and explain why they are not accurate.
Fifty percent of people over 85 years live in nursing homes. True or false?
Do changing private and public social roles affect the aging adult? How?
What does it mean to be dependent?
Socialization and being connected to others is not important to an aging adult. True or false?
What is meant by normal or successful aging?

Summary Tips

Be sensitive to clients' cultural, spiritual, and religious backgrounds.
Listening to individual wants and needs will build better relationships for better client care.
Help the home care client create opportunities for socialization and positive interactions with others.
Provide the client with a safe environment for sharing thoughts, concerns, and feelings by not passing judgment.
Encourage any client who is struggling to accept and cope with the aging process to seek help from a clergy person, doctor, social worker, or mental health professional.

Helpful Web Sites

Administration on Aging: http://www.aoa.gov
Information about Aging: American Association of Retired Persons (AARP) at http://www.aarp.org
American Psychological Association: http://www.apa.org/topics/topicaging.html

Suggested Reading

Cohen, Gene. (2001). *The creative age: Awakening human potential in the second half of life*. New York: HarperCollins. History, science, and true-life stories about human vitality and creative powers that come with age and experience.
Dass, Ram. (2001). *Still here: Embracing aging, changing, and dying*. New York: Penguin Group. A spiritual guide to all who are or will be old.

Pipher, Mary. (1999). *Another country: Navigating the emotional terrain of our elders.* New York: Penguin Putnam Inc. What elders experience, why there is trouble relating with them, and how to make the process of aging more pleasant for them and eventually ourselves.

Thomas, William. (2006). *In the arms of elders: A parable of wise leadership and community building.* Acton, MA: Vanderwyk and Burnham. The value of elders at the core of building community.

Aging at Home

2

In This Chapter, You Will Learn

1. The concepts and attitudes of caregiving

2. To identify services and trends of in-home care

3. The difference between Activities of Daily Living (ADLs) and Instrumental Activities of Daily Living (IADLs)

4. The advantages and disadvantages of home health and long-term care

Why This Matters

Understanding why and how the role of family caregiving has changed over the generations helps explain why there is the need for home care services. As the aging population increases, so does the demand for care services. Most people prefer to remain living in their own homes and fear moving to a nursing home even before they enter older adulthood, which has pushed the need for alternatives to long-term-care living facilities. The home care industry is expanding to meet the supply and demand of the older adult population through a variety of home care services. Home care providers are indispensable members of the home caregiving community.

Caregiving and Caregivers

Caregiving is the commonly used term for the practice of caring for an aged, infirmed, or disabled loved one, which can progress over a period of time or occur suddenly as the result of an accident or illness. The essence of caregiving implies the understanding of an individual's personality—likes, dislikes, habits, and nuances—that broadens a human relationship with focus on values, interests, and the potential of the person for whom care is being provided. Caring for another person is any combination of decision making for medical, social, and physical service needs, on an alternating or regular routine. Decisions are made daily, weekly, or monthly regarding intermittent, respite, or 24-hour care.

The faces of caregivers are parents, spouses, sons, daughters, friends, and neighbors. There is no age discrimination; the need to assume responsibility for another person can arise at any time in one's life. Many cultures have managed this family dynamic for generations. Traditionally, family members have provided for the personal needs of others and managed the issues that arise when caring for another with little to no relief from outside this network. Family systems continue to be an integral element for planning and providing care, though family structures and capacities are changing for several reasons, including but not limited to:

Family members are not living as physically near to each other as they once did. This distance has created the need for nonfamily members to provide care that was once considered a family responsibility.

The average life span at the start of the 20th century was 45 years, and 78 years at the turn of the 21st century (The President's Council on Bioethics, 2002). Advancements in medical technologies have lengthened the life span; more people are living longer with serious conditions that require regular attention and intervention.

Caregiving has historically been the responsibility of women in the family; in the 21st century, women account for nearly half of the U.S. workforce. The demands of caregiving challenge their availability for balancing family and work responsibilities and obligations.

High costs of hospitals; acute, subacute, and extended-care facilities have an impact on care decisions and provisions.

Caregiving responsibilities are being shared with outside support systems just in time for the increasing aging population propelled by the Baby Boomer Generation. This surge, coupled with changing family dynamics, is increasing the need for professional assistance and expanding job opportunities for trained care providers.

In the 21st century, caregiving is an evolving concept influenced by social, economic, and geographic issues that extend beyond the family system.

Social Issues

Caregiving needs are influencing the workplace, social institutions, public policy, and legislature. The National Family Caregivers Association (NFCA) has been instrumental in directing national attention to current and future federal policies that specifically impact family caregivers. (Federal legislation information—pending and passed—can be found by contacting state senators and representatives.) Government programs exist in which family caregivers are compensated for missed work time in order to provide direct care. Some employers will offer flexible work schedules to accommodate employees who are family caregivers. Workplace employee assistance programs assist in locating support networks and informational resources. Religious and nonprofit organizations offer workshops and training on caregiving skills, as well as provide referrals for support services.

Economic Issues

The rising costs of medications, treatments, hospitals, and care facilities have tremendous impact on care choices and practices. The Metropolitan Life Insurance Company Mature Market Institute (2007) produced survey results in September 2005 showing the average daily rate of a semiprivate room in a nursing home is $176.00, or $64,240 annually. The average hourly rate for companion care providers is $17.00, or $35,360 for a 52-week work year. When home care provisions are viable, they are clearly the more affordable option, which contributes to the economic planning of caregiving situations. There are other costs to the informal caregiver: phone expenses, travel time and expenses, and time missed at work. The psychological and emotional tolls of caregiving are just as significant.

Geographic Issues

Families are no longer living in as close proximity as they once did, which impacts how routines and decisions for care are determined. Out-of-town family members may not be readily available to assess the caregiving situation and may not be physically present to observe or provide supervision. The need for a person outside of the family system to give assistance may be necessary. Rapport and trust with formal caregivers is particularly important to out-of-town family members because they are not able to personally monitor the care recipient's needs or care provider's attendance.

Attitudes on Caregiving

Despite the degree of responsibility or time involved in the caregiving situation, family caregivers reflect on the changing roles and relationships that may require becoming a parent to the parent. Just as older adults can struggle with the psychology of aging, family members acting as caregivers contemplate the roles and responsibilities of caregiving. Emotionally, it can be difficult for family members to watch a loved one decline. At any sign of forgetfulness, family caregivers tend to worry that an aging parent has Alzheimer's disease or another dementia. The changing relationship often requires effort and patience to create the delicate balance of making decisions while maintaining the care recipient's independence and dignity. Ensuring that a care recipient is safe and satisfied with decisions that are made is not always simple or easy. Family members are conscious about their parents' happiness: if the parent is not happy, chances are the family will not be either. When a parent is unhappy with the direction of care, family caregivers may feel inept, which can lead to feelings of guilt. Money and financial resources to pay for care or daily living expenses are yet another concern for many. Family caregivers often feel obligated to help aging parents though may be limited by personal, family, and professional demands and responsibilities.

On top of relationship and financial issues, family caregivers also contemplate their own fears of aging and dying. Watching a parent or other loved one age reminds us that life is fragile and terminal. Any exposure to poor care through the health care system reinforces the fears of aging and illness. Observing hospital practices, medical technology, and measures of life support can be very frightening, practically forcing one to think of how they will want to be treated in end-of-life circumstances. Family members think about their own future when they visit a parent who lives in a nursing home where the roommate acts out inappropriately. These vulnerabilities deter some family members from becoming caregivers.

The unpleasant reality of caregiving is that it is portrayed as a burden, which impacts the way care is delivered and received. The business of the aging is to be sick and the business of caregiving is to be demanding. Society's stigma on caregiving can inhibit family members and nonfamily members from assuming the role of a caregiver. Stigma also affects the care recipient, who does not want to be viewed as needy or dependent. Additionally, care recipients are well aware of sacrifices family members may need to assume in order to become caregivers. As a result, care recipients feel guilty for needing the help and needing family members to make obligatory arrangements for them.

The Caregiving Community at Home

Family and friends, known as *informal caregivers* because they are typically not trained and may not be compensated for giving care, are usually the first to get involved with nonskilled care tasks when a family member or friend is in need. Several studies show that wives, daughters, and other female family members become the primary caregivers in these situations. It can be emotionally difficult and depressing for friend and family caregivers to watch a loved one in a deteriorated state. The informal caregiver may become unable to provide the necessary care, creating the need for outside assistance. The paid providers from a private business or home health or social service agency are known as *formal caregivers* and considerably benefit the informal caregiving system, which includes the home care recipient. Assistance from formal care providers offers emotional and physical support to informal caregivers, even if it is only to allow the caregiver much-needed time away from the caregiving situation. See Table 2.1 for statistical profiles of caregivers. Furthermore, formal care providers become emotional outlets to whom the care recipient will express feelings and worries, rather than add the perceived burden of emotional matters on informal caregivers. Formal systems of structured home care services have become the favored method for receiving care. Studies show that caregivers who use supportive services and respite care, and attend support groups or counseling, are able to provide care longer with greater satisfaction (Family Caregiver Alliance, n.d.-b).

2.1 Statistics of Caregiving

- Relationship of Caregiver to Care Recipient

Wife	13%
Husband	10%
Daughter	26%
Son	15%
Other Female Relative	17.5%
Other Male Relative	8.6%
Female Non-Relative	5.7%
Male Non-Relative	1.8%

- Female Caregivers — 63%
- Male Caregivers — 35%
- Relative Caregiver — 85%
- Friend/Neighbor — 15%
- Number of caregivers caring for those over 50 — 34 million
- Informal caregivers to those over 65 who need assistance with everyday activities — 5–7 million
- Adults in the community who depend on informal caregivers as their only source of help — 78%
- Adults in the community who use a combination of informal and formal caregiver assistance — 14%
- Adults in the community who use only formal caregivers — 8%

Note: From Family Caregiver Alliance (n.d.). http://www.caregiver.org/caregiver/jsp/content_node.jsp?nodeid=440

Home Care and Home Health Care

As more people of all ages are living with chronic conditions and debilitating illnesses, they are choosing to receive care in their own homes instead of in an institutional setting. This demand for both physical and social home care has increased the number of home health businesses and expanded the industry's service offerings. The growth in number and variety of home care services has helped to establish the credibility of the home health care industry. Home care agencies offer multidiscipline services by employing nurses, therapists, nurse aides, homemakers, and companions. Hospice care is also delivered in the home. Many medical treatments and care routines once provided only in a hospital or nursing home are now available at home. The industry's expansion has created informational service businesses from which care recipients, caregivers, and other providers seek information from professionals to guide them to appropriate resources and services. If financial resources are available and health-related issues are not compromised, home health care has become the preferred alternative.

What is home health care? It is any combination of physical, medical, mental, and social services brought to a person in the home rather than the care recipient going to a hospital, nursing home, or rehabilitation center. The choice of home care means hiring professionals and specialists to come into the home to offer care, as family members are unlikely trained or able to perform many treatments and routines. The number of hospital visits and length of time spent in a hospital are decreasing as more care recipients are choosing in-home and outpatient medical services and treatment options. The decision for care at home can delay the need for long-term-care placement.

There is a distinction between home health care and home care, which can be defined through two classifications: skilled and nonskilled care. Home health care implies the need for skilled services and home care attends to nonskilled care services.

Skilled care involves:

Nursing services
Medical treatments and monitoring
Medication routines
Physical or occupational therapies

Nonskilled care is broad, encompassing:

Personal care routines, such as bathing, dressing, and eating
Errand running
Household maintenance tasks
Homemaking and meal preparation
Social Services, to offer support, education, and information of community
    resources
Supervision of the home caregiving situation

A general rule of thumb is that skilled care provides aid with Activities of Daily Living and nonskilled care is assistance with Instrumental Activities of Daily Living.

Activities of Daily Living (ADLs) and Instrumental Activities of Daily Living (IADLs)

In home care, home health care, and nursing home care, care recipients' capabilities are evaluated to determine functioning status. Nurses, social workers, and physical and occupational therapists assess a person through observation and a series of physical and cognitive evaluations. These assessments measure the person's ability to perform personal care routines, known as Activities of Daily Living, as well as the ability to complete everyday tasks done throughout all ages and stages of life, called Instrumental Activities of Daily Living. These same health care professionals then make necessary referrals for service provisions. Informal caregivers may also notice the need for assistance in these areas and arrange for services without assistance from health care professionals.

Activities of Daily Living are:

Bathing
Toileting
Dressing
Transfers
Feeding
Functional mobility programs
Brushing teeth
Other personal hygiene care

Instrumental Activities of Daily Living are:

Bill paying
Appointment scheduling
Money management
Meal preparation
Grocery shopping
Other shopping
Errand running
Making telephone calls
Household maintenance
Light house cleaning
Laundry
Home organization
Pet care
Medication routines
Recreational opportunities
Transportation/travel

Home health care providers offer services based on these Instrumental/Activities of Daily Living. Depending on the area of need, the care providers who deliver service may or may not need to be licensed or certified by a body of oversight, such as a state health department. For example, providing care with Activities of Daily Living usually requires a certified nursing assistant or nurse while a care provider who runs errands and offers companionship (IADLs) may not need to be certified. This area of the home care industry is booming with business start-ups as hired care providers are replacing family, friends, and neighbors to offer assistance with Instrumental Activities of Daily Living.

Choosing Home Care

Home care options are diverse and plentiful whether services are provided by a hired individual or through a home health care agency. It should be noted that healthy older adults choose to employ people to provide home-assistance services. As people age and their wants and needs change, there can be a natural progression to downsize and simplify life. Able-bodied older adults may hire help with managing household tasks, such as bill paying, preparing meals, transportation, and housekeeping. Assistance with these tasks may be just enough support to keep the individual living independently in their own home.

Care recipients or family caregivers can choose from the following typical services:

Companion
Homemaking
Errand running
Home and personal chores
Personal care
Nursing
Medical equipment and supplies
Respite care
Home-delivered meals
Transportation
Money management
Counseling

An explanation of these home care services is offered below.

Companions and Homemakers

Companions are involved in caregiving situations to provide company and friendship to care recipients. In some circumstances, a companion may run errands or provide transportation. Homemakers tend to household chores and cleaning routines that have become difficult or time consuming for care recipients. The responsibilities of companions and homemakers often overlap depending on the individual or agency job description. Typical responsibilities are:

Conversation and companionship
Medication reminders
Light housekeeping
Meal planning and preparation
Grocery shopping

Taking out the garbage
Scheduling appointments
Recreational activities
Coordinating home maintenance routines
Supervision of home and personal needs

Nurse Aides and Nurses

Nurse aides may also offer companion and homemaking services, though they primarily provide assistance with bathing, dressing, and other personal care routines. Nurses who make home visits are often dependent on the paying source. Care recipients' needs and conditions shape service offerings; diagnoses and insurance policies have an effect on home care service delivery. Home care provisions can be restricted when insurance, including Medicare, pays for the services. If a home care recipient is paying with private money, service offerings and schedules are flexible and only limited by his or her financial resources.

Medical Equipment and Supplies

Typically, physical and occupational therapists or nurses complete evaluations and make recommendations for necessary equipment. Common medical equipment and supplies range from canes, grabbers, elevated commode seats, and bedside toilets to walkers, lift chairs, electric wheelchairs, and hospital beds. Some products can be easily purchased over the counter and paid for with private money. Insurance will cover the cost of certain products with a doctor's order. There are multiple ways of acquiring medical equipment and supplies, depending on what type of product is needed. Home deliveries are available or products can be picked up from a medical supply store.

Respite Care

The demands of caring for a loved one influence emotional, social, and work attitudes and activities. The opportunity for relief from a caregiving situation is ideal. Respite care is intended to provide relief for primary or family caregivers, and implies that the care recipient will remain in the current living situation with temporary adjustments. The typical form of respite care is the hiring of formal or informal care providers who come into the home to stay with the care recipient for a designated period of time. This allows the primary or family caregivers to take a break from the responsibilities of caregiving. Or, the care recipient might be placed in a facility for a short-term, temporary stay while family caregivers take time away from the caregiving situation.

Home-Delivered Meals

Home-delivered meals are available, most commonly through the Meals on Wheels program. Consult the yellow pages, talk with an agency social worker, or contact the Area Agency on Aging to learn more about the options in your area.

Transportation

There is a growing need for transportation services for the elderly and disabled. Services vary depending on needs. Some care recipients no longer have driving privileges but are physically capable of getting in and out of a car. Other care recipients have physical restrictions that prohibit driving and can also make transferring in and out of a car difficult. Transportation needs may be as simple as taking the care recipient to a doctor's appointment, grocery store, or pharmacy. Individuals, taxicabs, or private transportation companies are most widely used in these situations. Many cities and towns have public transportation services for qualified seniors and disabled persons. Private companies exist to provide specialized transportation services to people in wheelchairs or with other adaptive equipment who have difficulty using a personal car or taxicab. To learn about transportation services in your area, contact the Area Agency on Aging or check the local yellow pages.

Money Management

Attorneys and accountants oversee clients' financial planning and tax preparations, generally on an annual basis. Other professionals specifically assist senior clients with weekly and monthly money management. Individuals and agencies may offer monthly bill pay assistance that can include sitting with a client to review and pay routine household bills. Additionally, there are professionals who specifically manage Medicare, insurance, and medical claims.

Counseling

Mental health professionals and case managers, usually from community-based treatment centers, are providing home counseling treatments and services. Most counselors, psychologists, and psychiatrists require that the client come to the professional's office; with less frequency, they will make house visits. Counseling services in the home could become readily available as the needs of the aging population change and expand.

Community-Based Services

In addition to services available in the home, there are other community resources that should not be overlooked. Senior centers and adult day care centers are additional levels of service that exist to help a person stay in their home instead of moving into a nursing home or other long-term-care facility. These two options offer socialization, stimulation, and supervision for the client who does not need 24-hour care.

Senior Centers

Typically, senior centers serve residents of neighborhoods and areas local to the center. The goal of a senior center is to provide socialization and activities for seniors who live in the community. Participants are usually high functioning, needing little to no physical assistance with mobility, ADLs, and IADLs. Many senior centers are social outlets; programming varies by center, though it generally includes arts and crafts, dance, exercise, games and cards, and educational programs. Because they are considered social outlets, lunches are often available, and minimal nursing services (i.e., blood pressure checks) may be offered. Attendees can show up for part of or the entire day; transportation services to and from the center may or may not be available. Every senior center is different; it is recommended to tour the center and ask plenty of questions.

Adult Day Care

Day care is very similar to senior centers in that it is a day program that provides activities and stimulation, and more often than not nursing services are offered. Adult day care clients usually require more supervision and assistance with Activities of Daily Living. Many adult day care clients live in the community independently, or with a spouse or other family member. Transportation to and from the center is usually available. As with senior centers, adult day care centers vary from city to city and state to state. It is recommended to tour the facility and ask plenty of questions.

The Home Care Industry

The advantages and benefits of care at home are the reasons the home health industry has become so large and the preferred choice in health care options. The increased need for home health care has opened new job and career opportunities. The home health care industry is one of the fastest growing employment markets. The U.S. Bureau of Labor Statistics reports over 13,000 people employed in the health care industry in 2004, and employment in this industry will increase, reaching over 27,000 by 2014 (U.S. Bureau of Labor Statistics, 2007). Specifically, home health aides, including those self-employed, will increase more than 55% by 2014. According to the U.S. Bureau of Labor Statistics, home health employment opportunities are expected to grow more than 25% through the year 2014 for several reasons. The increased number of aged persons will create the demand for more health care workers. The acceptance that many treatments are more effective in familiar settings will increase home-based treatment options. Technological advancement of medical equipment and treatments is progressing home care services and delivery. In addition, costs for home care are more often than not less than hospitals and nursing facilities. (See Table 2.2.)

The Family Caregiver Alliance (n.d.-a) reports that a skilled-nursing facility averages four times more in expenses than does paid, in-home care within the community. The Family Caregiver Alliance (n.d.-a) also reports the following:

The 85 years and older age group is one of the largest growing population segments. By 2050, the number of persons 85 and older is expected to be 19.4 million.

27 million people will be using long-term-care services in various settings by the year 2050 (e.g., at home, residential care such as assisted living, or skilled-nursing facilities).

2.2 Comparison of Home Care and Nursing Home Costs

Home care	Percentage/number of
• 2002 care in the community costs	$36.1 billion
• By 2050, the number of individuals using long-term-care services at home, assisted living, or skilled-nursing facilities will likely double	13 million using services in 2000 will rise to 27 million people
• People who need long-term care who live at home or in community settings, not in institutions	79%
Nursing home/extended care	
• 2002 nursing home costs	$103.2 billion
• 2002 public and private spending on long-term-care services	exceeded $180 billion
• Out-of-pocket expenses paid by individual or family	$37.2 billion, or 21%
• Annual (2004) rate for private room	$70,080
• Annual (2004) rate for semiprivate room	$61,685
• People living in nursing homes (2002)	1,458,000

Note: From http://www.caregiver.org/caregiver/jsp/content_node.jsp?nodeid=440

The Aging Population

Death rates have been declining since the middle of the 20th century, while life expectancy rates have been on the rise. In 1999, the life expectancy for a male was 74; in 2025, the expectancy age is 76.5 (Russell, 2000). For females, the life expectancy rate in 1999 was 79; in 2025, it is expected to be 82.6 (Russell, 2000). Additional demographics by age and gender are provided in Table 2.3 as retrieved from the U.S. Census Bureau (2004) Web site.

The Baby Boomer Generation

This population gets its designation based on the time period in which they were born. The Baby Boomer Generation is simply defined as those born between the years of 1946 and 1964; at the end of World War II in 1945 the soldiers returned home, and there was an increase in births during the following 18 years. Research indicates over 75 million American babies were born during this 18-year period, making up nearly 30% of the current population. Obviously,

2.3 Population Estimates and Projections of the U.S. by Age, 2000–2050

Total population (in thousands)

	2000	2010	2020	2030	2040	2050
65–84	30,794	34,120	47,363	61,850	64,640	65,844
	10.90%	11.00%	14.10%	17.00%	16.50%	15.70%
85+	4,267	6,123	7,269	9,603	15,409	20,861
	1.50%	2.00%	2.20%	2.60%	3.90%	5.00%
Male 65–84	9.50%	9.90%	12.90%	15.70%	15.30%	14.80%
85+	9.00%	1.30%	1.50%	1.90%	2.90%	3.80%
Female 65–84	12.20%	12.10%	15.20%	18.30%	17.60%	16.50%
85+	2.10%	2.70%	2.90%	3.40%	4.90%	6.10%

Note: From http://www.census.gov/ipc/www/usinterimproj/natprojtab02a.pdf

the majority of these people will age and become senior citizens. According to the Administration on Aging (2007), 12% percent of the population were persons 65 years and older in 2002; by 2030, that same demographic will reach nearly 25%, more than twice the number from 2002. The following chart takes a closer look at the length of time the Baby Boomer Generation will be the aged population.

2.4 Year reaching

Born in	65 years	80 years
1946	2011	2026
1964	2029	2044

The Baby Boomer Generation will reach 65 years in 2011 and 80 years in 2026 (see Table 2.4). Children born in the last year of the Baby Boomer Generation, 1964, will turn 65 years in 2029 and 80 years in 2044. This visual aid shows us that the Baby Boomers will be the aging population from 2011 through 2044, which does not even consider those who live longer than 80 years! We can also see that when the earliest Baby Boomers reach 80 in 2026, the youngest of the Baby Boomers will be reaching 65 in less than 5 years. This entire 33-year period, which will have a highly populated aging demographic that will likely need many types of health care services, will be a busy time for the health care industry.

Rights for the Home Care Client

In July 1999, the U.S. Supreme Court decided that persons with disabilities have the right to receive care in the home rather than being placed in a nursing home or other institution. This is known as the Olmstead Decision. As a result, state and national government-funded programs that serve the aging population and those with disabilities will create more community-based options, resources, and solutions for long-term-care needs as well as alternatives to nursing home placement. Additional programs and service offerings will grow over time to continually meet the needs of the aging population. Further, these efforts will reinforce the need and desire for in-home care as an alternative to nursing home placement, thereby supporting the home health care service industry.

We frequently hear about "client rights" in the health care industry. What does this mean? Client rights, across industry lines, are essentially a set of guidelines established to ensure that a client is entitled to express needs and preferences pertaining to service delivery. There are moral, civil, constitutional, and legal rights to be upheld that do not end because of age. For example, it is a legal right for an American to drive at the age of 16 and continue to drive, regardless of age, as long as the person is able to fulfill the responsibilities for safe driving.

The National Association for Home Care & Hospice (NAHC) has created a model Bill of Rights for home health care recipients based on current federal laws (see Tip 2.1). It is a federal law that all home care recipients are informed of their patient rights.

Tip 2.1

Clients Have the Right to . . .

Choose care providers
Be fully informed of all rights and responsibilities by the home care provider
Appropriate and professional care in accordance with physicians' orders
Receive a timely response from the agency to request for service

Be admitted for service only if the agency has the ability to provide safe, professional care at the level of intensity needed

Receive reasonable continuity of care

Receive information necessary to give informed consent prior to the start of any treatment or procedure

Be advised of any change in the plan of care, before the change is made

Refuse treatment within the confines of the law and to be informed of the consequences of his or her action

Be informed of his or her rights under state law to formulate advance directives

Have health care providers comply with advance directives in accordance with state law requirements

Be informed within reasonable time of anticipated termination of service or plans for transfer to another agency

Be fully informed of agency policies and charges for services, including eligibility for third-party reimbursements

Be referred elsewhere, if denied service solely on his or her inability to pay

Voice grievances and suggest changes in service or staff without fear of restraint or discrimination

A fair hearing for any individual to whom any service has been denied, reduced, or terminated, or who is otherwise aggrieved by agency action. The fair hearing procedure shall be set forth by each agency as appropriate to the unique patient situation (i.e., funding source, level of care, diagnosis)

Be informed of what to do in the event of an emergency

Reproduced with the express and limited permission of the National Association for Home Care & Hospice. All rights reserved.

The Eden Alternative at Home

The delivery of home care services is loosely structured on the idea of meeting personalized needs of care recipients through one-on-one attention without a description of what quality service provisions are or how they can be accomplished. Care providers' attitudes and perceptions toward aged adults and the aging process will influence the style and manner in which he or she gives care. The Eden Alternative is a noteworthy project that was established to change the attitudes and perceptions of aging and how to care for the aged. The principles and practices of the Eden Alternative seek to offer a compassionate approach to caring for the aging.

The Eden Alternative was designed by Dr. William Thomas, a Harvard-educated physician and board-certified geriatrician, to combat what are considered the three plagues of life—loneliness, helplessness, and boredom

(Eden Alternative, 2007c). The concept is simple: The aging process should be managed as another stage of growth and development. The 10 guiding principles of the Eden Alternative (2007b) are:

1. The three plaques of loneliness, helplessness, and boredom account for the bulk of suffering among our elders.
2. An Elder-centered community commits to creating a Human Habitat where life revolves around close and continuing contact with plants, animals, and children. These relationships provide the young and old alike with a pathway to a life worth living.
3. Loving companionship is the antidote to loneliness. Elders deserve easy access to human and animal companionship.
4. An Elder-centered community creates opportunity to give as well as receive care. This is the antidote to helplessness.
5. An Elder-centered community imbues daily life with variety and spontaneity by creating an environment in which unexpected and unpredictable interactions and happenings can take place. This is the antidote to boredom.
6. Meaningless activity corrodes the human spirit. The opportunity to do things we find meaningful is essential to human health.
7. Medical treatment should be the servant of genuine human caring, never its master.
8. An Elder-centered community honors its Elders by de-emphasizing top-down bureaucratic authority, seeking instead to place the maximum possible decision making authority into the hands of the Elders or into the hands of those closest to them.
9. Creating an Elder-centered community is a never-ending process. Human growth must never be separated from human life.
10. Wise leadership is the lifeblood of any struggle against the three plagues. For this, there can be no substitute.

Eden at Home aims to improve the quality of life for those receiving home care and community-based services. Eden at Home emphasizes that a home is not only the living environment; to a greater extent, a home is an elder's community and world, and the manner in which the aging adult integrates these aspects of life (Eden Alternative, 2007d). The goal of Eden at Home is to create the most positive experience of older adulthood possible through the application of four main ideas (Eden Alternative, 2007d):

1. Elders have legacies to share with their loved ones and community.
2. Meaningful care nurtures the human spirit as well as the human body by recognizing, celebrating, and nurturing each individual's unique capacity for growth.
3. The elder, or care receiver, is an active participant in his or her own care plan; thus, a care partner.
4. Elderhood is honored as a valued phase of human development rather than merely the decline of life.

The Eden Alternative is also working to change the culture of long-term-care organizations (Eden Alternative, 2007c). At the center of the Eden Alternative's principles is to keep elders participating in care decisions. Facilities that make use of the Eden Alternative involve residents in organizational planning to enhance service offerings, as well as encourage individuals to make personal health care decisions. Whether in the community, at home, or in a long-term-care setting, care providers can apply the principles and philosophy of the Eden concept to offer excellent service. Quality care providers understand and accept a care recipient for the person that he or she has become as an older adult. This appreciation and acknowledgment validates care recipients' self-confidence, which is necessary for successful growth in the aging process. Without recognition or appropriate support, aging adults can feel lonely and out of touch. Even at home, caregiving situations can feel like institutions when (Eden Alternative, 2007d)

Care partners and care receivers are not empowered
Spontaneity and variety are absent from daily life
Diversity and access to companionship are limited
There are no opportunities to give as well as receive
The focus of the care revolves solely around the physical body
Teamwork is not utilized by care partners to meet challenges
The emphasis is placed on the idea of treatment and task-doing rather than caregiving

The importance of the Eden concept at home or in a facility is, in the least, two-fold. First, that care providers—ideally, the general society—*embrace* the idea of "Elderhood" (Eden Alternative, 2007d). According to the Eden Alternative (2007d) Web site, Dr. Thomas suggests that "acknowledging and embracing the idea of Elder-richness and strengthening the exchange between the generations can improve quality of life for all ages." Second, the Eden Alternative philosophy suggests what individuals need that will support growth during the aging process. Eden at Home seeks to integrate elders back into their physical and social communities; by embracing elderhood, this is possible.

Summary

The act of caregiving is about good decision making: balancing judgments and safety concerns while preserving the others' dignity and independence. Activities of caregiving include: coordinating home care services, monitoring care and routines in the home or a facility, giving direct care, supervising medications, managing financial and legal matters, providing transportation, encouraging social and recreational stimulation, and offering emotional support. There are as many aspects of caregiving as there are caregiving situations.
The trend for home health care and community-based services is on the rise. The number of businesses established to offer home health care services is expanding along with the diverse types of in-home service offerings. Opportunities in home health employment are expected to grow more than 25% through the year 2014. Consumers are choosing home health care services over

long-term-care placement. The costs of care at home are considerably less than institutional costs, which affect care decisions. Studies show that care recipients respond better to care in a familiar, homelike setting.

Home care recipients have legal rights to quality care and to direct their course of care as able. It makes good sense to know an agency's protocol for ensuring these legal rights are fulfilled.

The Eden Alternative is a noteworthy project that was established to change the attitudes and perceptions of aging and caring for the aged. Efforts toward eliminating loneliness, helplessness, and boredom in extended-care facilities and in the home are significant contributions to embracing elderhood.

Questions

What types of home care services are available?

Why are the roles and responsibilities of a caregiver considered burdensome?

What is the difference between formal and informal caregivers?

Why is it becoming more common for families to use formal caregivers?

Why are consumers choosing home health services over placement in a facility?

What is the impact of the Baby Boomer Generation on the aging population?

Name two types of community-based services for senior citizens.

What is a significant difference between senior centers and adult day care centers?

What should happen when clients' rights are not being upheld?

What are the three plagues of life in a care facility, according to the Eden Alternative?

Summary Tips

Learn the types of home care services available and when they're appropriate for particular client situations.

Be understanding and suspend judgment of families' need for formal caregivers when caring for their elder loved one; caring for a loved one can be emotionally challenging.

To learn about current legislative issues and trends pertaining to home care, visit the Web sites of organizations such as the National Council for Home Care & Hospice, the National Family Caregiver Alliance, the Centers for Medicare and Medicaid, and the Administration on Aging.

Helpful Web Sites

To locate your state senators: United States Senate, http://www.senate.gov

To locate your state representative: United States House of Representatives http://www.house.gov

Caregiving information, education, trends and statistics:

Family Caregiver Alliance/National Center on Caregiving: http://www.caregiver.org

National Family Caregivers Association: http://www.nfcacares.org

National Association for Home Care and Hospice: http://www.nahc.org

U.S. Administration on Aging: http://www.aoa.gov

Employment and Jobs in Caregiving and Home Health Care: Bureau of Labor Statistics, http://stats.bls.gov/bls/occupation.htm

Olmstead Decision: http://www.ltcombudsman.org

AARP (American Association of Retired Persons): http://www.research.aarp.org

The Eden Alternative: http://www.edenalt.org

Suggested Reading

Baker, Beth. (2007). *Old age in a new age: The promise of transformative nursing homes.* Nashville, TN: Vanderbilt University Press. A personal journey into more than two dozen nursing homes considered the best places in America for elders to live.

Caputo, Richard (Ed.). (2005). *Challenges of aging on U.S. families: Policy and practice implications.* Philadelphia, PA: Haworth Press. Trends, issues, and the impact the aging baby boomer generation will have on their families and American society.

Dimidjian, Victoria Jean. (2004). *Journeying east: Conversations of aging and dying.* Rocklin, CA: Parallax Press. Thoughts on aging and the end-of-life process by spiritual leaders.

Kiernan, Stephen. (2006). *Last rights: Rescuing the end of life from the medical system.* New York: St. Martin's Press. Research and stories about end-of-life care and decision making.

Winokur, Juli. (2003). *Aging in America: The years ahead.* New York: PowerHouse Books. Challenges of the growing aging population in American society.

The Companion Home Care Provider

3

In This Chapter, You Will Learn

1. Roles and responsibilities of the nonmedical home care provider

2. How to document observations and client activities

3. Regularly used medical terminology abbreviations

4. The value of establishing goals and objectives

5. Suggestions for relieving stress

Why This Matters

Every job comes with a description that defines its tasks and responsibilities. Beyond the employer's expectations, there is personal responsibility to make oneself a better employee who offers quality in work performance. Agency policies and procedures are required knowledge, while there is also a body of unspoken and implied information that is learned through personal and professional experiences. Excellent home care providers strive to reach personal and work-related goals that advance service improvement. This chapter speaks to the specialized personal and professional responsibilities of companions and nonmedical home care providers.

The Companion

Companions have become a basic component of home care services, whether family members live nearby or not. A person may be hired as a companion because there are no family members, family is not available (due to time, distance, or other demands), or the family members do not have the necessary skills and training or emotional capability. Families may ask a companion to act as another set of eyes because the recipient needs to have a "friend" outside of the family system. A companion is an advocate who gathers information and reports to managers, supervisors, and directly with family caregivers. The need to have a person regularly monitor, supervise, and provide support services to a care recipient in the home or in a facility is becoming recognized as a practical, affordable comfort or a necessity that can delay the decision and need for assisted living or extended-care-facility placement.

Companions and nonmedical home care providers assist with the Instrumental Activities of Daily Living (IADLs). Nonmedical home care providers should not perform duties they are not trained to do; they are not always licensed or certified nursing assistants, who typically provide assistance with Activities of Daily Living (ADLs). Changes in a client's self-performance are frequently signs of a decreased ability to maintain usual self-care routines and the incapability to manage general responsibilities. A care recipient's ability to perform IADLs and ADLs is used to measure functioning levels. It is the noticeable changes in IADLs or ADLs that convince family members, friends, and others of the need for in-home help or alternative living arrangements. (See the following case study about "Jane.")

Home care agencies, including hospice, have expanded services and staff with the option of companion care. An agency that provides skilled-nursing services, such as nursing or medical procedures and physical therapy, is usually Medicare certified, which means that Medicare reimburses the agency a portion or the full amount for the cost of service. Companion care and nonmedical support services are not eligible for Medicare's reimbursement, and payment comes directly from the care recipient.

Companions and care providers give quality of life to their care recipients. Friendships are formed because of the amount of time care providers spend providing personal attention to care recipients. A care recipient's trust in the care provider is the essential component of a successful care recipient–care provider relationship. Trust is more than the assurance that a care provider will appear when expected and not remove items from the home; it is the faith that excellent care will be offered. Care providers are the voices that advocate care recipients' wants and needs while acting as their eyes, ears, and even their memory. The essence of this trust allows the care provider in to the position of judgment, which creates intimacy—the true spirit of connecting with another human being. They are then able to form deeper relationships and understand perceptions from the care recipient's viewpoint. Care providers must be attentive and observant to the range of needs for nutrition, activity, rest, safety, emotional well-being, and medical attention (see Tip 3.1). A quality care provider focuses on client abilities and strengths, paying attention to what the client is able to accomplish rather than what tasks he or she is not able to complete. Quality

Case Study

Jane, 80 years old, is high functioning with intact cognitive skills and independent in terms of decision making. Her physical abilities are severely limited by arthritis and osteoporosis. A recent fall resulted in a broken hip and collarbone; with limited mobility and physical restrictions, she moved into independent living. Jane's poor physical condition lengthens her daily routines and habits: Getting dressed can take as long as 2 hours, brushing and styling her hair takes an hour, and fixing a piece of toast—her preferred breakfast—can take 25 minutes.

Jane had been a journalist and hoped to continue writing in retirement. She had close relationships with friends, her children, and her grandchildren, and needed to keep regular contact; she felt a strong sense of self-worth by being available to them.

Jane's use of a cleaning service continued to help in the new living situation. She was urged by her daughter to also hire a companion to assist with noncleaning household tasks that had become time consuming and burdensome for Jane to complete on her own. Jane hired Eva, who completed these necessary tasks and afforded Jane the time she needed to tend to her personal care routines and other pursuits; without this assistance, Jane did not have enough time or energy in a day to maintain her quality of life.

As Jane's companion, Eva performed the following duties to alleviate Jane's workload:

Filled out checks weekly and monthly for Jane to sign
Set up bill pay through her online banking services
Traveled to the bank to cash checks and make deposits
Took Jane shopping as requested, or shopped for her
Took weekly trips to the drug and grocery stores for needed items
Scheduled doctor, dentist, acupuncture, and other appointments as needed
Drove Jane to appointments and picked up medical records from doctors
Helped with home office organization and filing
Made frequent contact with professionals, such as nurse, banker, attorney, pharmacist, and tax preparer

As Eva managed routine household maintenance, organization, and support services, Jane had the time and energy to maintain relationships and pursue her interests. Jane did not have to move to assisted living and was able to remain independent in her apartment.

care providers encourage efforts toward productive actions, which can build client motivation and self-confidence and, ultimately, dignity and independence. They provide meaningful experiences for the care recipient by creating a pleasant environment and demonstrating that they enjoy their work.

For the entrepreneurial type, providing nonmedical support services such as companion care and errand running has become a leading start-up idea for home-based businesses. Many states do not require a license to provide companion care, which has expanded the number of providers and business ventures (formal and informal structures) in the industry. It is not possible to determine the number of people providing companion and nonmedical support services due to the lack of licensing and certification requirements for companion care.

Tip 3.1

Thoughtful Assistance

Dressing is usually considered an ADL, though there may be times that a companion will need to assist the home care client with getting dressed, possibly due to an episode of incontinence, a food-spill accident, or the client's inability to get him/herself dressed before the companion's visit. Getting dressed can be physically challenging for some care recipients because of problems with fine or gross motor skills, while for others the dressing process is difficult due to impaired judgment or decision making. A companion can assist by using the following approaches:

Be patient. Encourage the care recipient to do as much possible on his or her own to promote independence and self-sufficiency. Allow the care recipient plenty of time to complete the task even if you could do it more quickly. Do not rush the care recipient, which could increase frustration and decrease his or her self-esteem. When it is obvious that the care recipient is unable to finish the task successfully, ask the care recipient if he or she is willing to accept help, and then provide assistance.

Minimize confusion. Offer only two or three choices, particularly if the care recipient is cognitively impaired or has difficulty making good decisions. For example, suggest the red or blue blouse, but do not overwhelm the care recipient with choices by also offering yellow, brown, and orange shirts. Consider if a mismatched outfit is important: Is it worth the attention if the end result will only escalate tension, anxiety, and frustration? Do help the care recipient choose weather-appropriate fabrics and outfits.

Keep it simple. Communicate through step-by-step instructions and be specific, especially when working with cognitively impaired persons. Demonstrating the intended action or behavior can be helpful. For instance, say "button the shirt" and demonstrate by buttoning one hole, rather than simply saying "get dressed." Keep in mind that getting dressed is an activity that uses cognitive and motor skills. A care recipient can feel a sense of accomplishment and pride by completing this task independently or with minimal assistance.

Case Study

Betty was a resident in independent living. She relinquished her driver's license due to Alzheimer's disease but began riding a bicycle as means for transportation. Sometimes she rode it 4 miles to church, though mostly she rode to the local market. For recreation, she took bike rides to search for aluminum cans that she took to be recycled weekly. Occasionally she would need light bicycle maintenance such as seat adjustments and remounting of the chain. Her companion was not prepared to be a bicycle mechanic but learned some simple repairs to make bike riding possible for Betty!

Roles and Responsibilities

A *role* means the position of a care provider, which is represented through the responsibilities of duties, obligations, and accountability for the purpose of caregiving. The roles and responsibilities of companion home care providers are to:

Roles

Examine safety issues and potential concerns
Supervise household maintenance and protection
Monitor nutrition, especially with restricted diets
Supervise medical/health conditions, chronic and acute
Monitor mental and cognitive functioning
Look for opportunities that enhance quality of life
Communicate client needs and concerns with family members or other persons involved in planning or decision making

In addition, a companion care provider should look tidy and neat, with conservative clothes, perfume, makeup, and jewelry. Good personal hygiene reflects upon the care that will be offered to the care recipient.

Responsibilities

Reliable attendance
Honesty, trustworthiness, and good judgment
Efficiency, flexibility, cooperativeness, and friendliness
Attentiveness to the client and home/living situation
Provide determined care requests by client and family
Maintain clients' dignity through home care patient bill of rights

Maintain quality of home life through home maintenance, organization, and chores

Promote safety in the home

Add quality of life through stimulating, recreational activities

Another important responsibility of a companion is to document and report observations to others involved in care provisions, especially changes in behavior and decline in functioning. Home health agency companions should report to managers, supervisors, nurses, or social workers. They must be sure to understand the organizational structure and follow the agency's policies and procedures for reporting. If the companion has been hired privately by the family or is a self-employed companion, establish one contact person to relay the information. A companion may communicate with other family members, though one contact person eliminates confusion and the question, "Did I remember to tell all four family members about the doctor's appointment next Wednesday?" The contact through one person allows more time to be spent with the client.

E-mail Correspondence

Joe began sending daily reports to his care recipients' family members through e-mail. For his client with Alzheimer's disease, in assisted living, Joe sent an e-mail to the client's brother, children, grandchildren, and a childhood friend. Joe reported their outings, recreational events, conversations, and his interactions with facility staff on a daily basis. This method of communication kept the out-of-town family members up to date about day-to-day care routines and the status of mom's disease progression. The frequent communication kept all members up to date on situations, which enhanced their decision making for mom.

Reporting can be tricky, particularly when a care provider is balancing the care recipient's need for privacy and independence while maintaining rapport with the care recipient and a realistic portrayal of the caregiving situation. Use good judgment when deciding on what information to share; matters of health and safety concerns should be addressed immediately. By using a nonjudgmental approach and focusing on problem solving, many issues can be discussed directly with the client, which contributes to relationship building with the care recipient. (More information on effective communication can be found in chapter 4, "Interpersonal Skills and Communications.")

Quality companion care should have some method of documentation; forms may vary, but there is little variation in content for recording observations. Often, these are carbon-copy forms that act as time sheets and are submitted to agency supervisors, mailed to family members, or even left in the home as confirmation that the companion was present. A sample form that contains subject matter to consider and observe for the documenting of daily activities and behaviors is offered in Figure 3.1 (see also Tip 3.2). (Both ADLs and IADLs are included in this example; complete as appropriate to job performance duties.)

3.1

Sample documentation form of daily activity log

Daily Activity Log

Client: _____   Date: _____

Time In: _____   Time out: _____   Mileage: _____

Meal Preparation: Diet Needs & Restrictions:
_____

Breakfast _____   _____
Lunch _____   Comments _____
Dinner _____   _____

IADL's	**ADL's**	**Other Assistance**
☐ bill pay assistance	☐ bathing	_____
☐ telephone assistance	☐ dressing	_____
☐ household maintenance	☐ ambulation program	_____
☐ pet care	☐ toileting	_____
☐ laundry	☐ feeding	_____
☐ cleaning	☐ personal hygiene	_____

Errands/Transportation: ☐ with client   ☐ without client

☐ grocery   ☐ drug store/Rx pick up   ☐ other shopping _____

☐ other _____
_____
_____

Recreation/Outings: _____
_____
_____

Upcoming Appointments

Dr, DDS, Hair, Other	Date	Time	Transportation
1.			
2.			
3.			
4.			

Cognitive or Behavior Changes (ST/LT memory, decision-making skills, vision/hearing/speech, mood)

Tip 3.2

Common Abbreviations in Health Care

Companions and other home care providers should be familiar with abbreviations used by health care professionals in order to better understand the medical situation and course of treatment.

AD: Alzheimer's disease
ADL: Activities of Daily Living
AFO: ankle-foot orthosis (swelling)
ASHD: arteriosclerotic heart disease
BC: blood culture
BID: 2 times per day
BP: blood pressure
BRP: bathroom privileges
BS: blood sugar
CA: cancer/carcinoma
CABG: coronary artery bypass graft
CBC: complete blood count
CCU: coronary care unit
CHF: congestive heart failure
CMS: Centers for Medicare and Medicaid Services
CNA: certified nurse aid
COPD: chronic obstructive pulmonary disease
CPR: cardiopulmonary resuscitation
CVA: cerebral vascular accident
CVD: cerebral vascular disease
DM: diabetes mellitus
DME: durable medical equipment
DNR: do not resuscitate
DPOA: durable power of attorney
DRG: diagnostic related group
EEG: electroencephalogram (recording of the brain's electrical activity)
EKG: electrocardiogram (recording of the heart's electrical activity)
ERS: emergency response system
FPG: fasting plasma glucose test (a test used to diagnose pre-diabetes or diabetes)
FX: fracture
HHA: home health agency or home health aid
HS: hour of sleep
IADL: Instrumental Activities of Daily Living
I & O: intake and output (record of food and beverage intake and elimination)
ICU: intensive care unit
INF: intermediate nursing facility
IV: intravenous line (to drip fluids into the bloodstream)

LOC: loss of consciousness or level of care
NPO: nothing by mouth
NSAID: nonsteroid anti-inflammatory drug
OBS: organic brain syndrome
OR: operating room
OT: occupational therapist
PCA: personal care aid
PO: by mouth
POC: plan of care (nursing home resident care plan or meeting to review care plan)
PRN: medications or treatments administered on as-needed basis
PRO: peer review organization (to monitor quality of Medicare and Medicaid)
PT: physical therapist
QID: 4 times per day
RBC: red blood count
ROM: range of motion
RR: respiratory rate
RT: recreational therapy
SOB: shortness of breath
SNF: skilled-nursing facility
TIA: transient ischemic attack
TID: 3 times per day
TPR: temperature, pulse, respiration (vital statistics)
TX: treatment
U/A: urine analysis
WBC: white blood count
WNL: within normal limit

Goals and Objectives

Goals describe the desired results and outcomes of a given project or program. The goal of caregiving is straightforward: to assist with and make decisions that maintain or improve the physical, mental, and social well-being of another person. The goal of companion care is to keep a client safe with the best quality of life offerings possible in their surroundings of choice. An objective is a specific action that is consistent with the goal. To accomplish any goal, clearly stated objectives must be identified and pursued. Often, more than one objective is stated for each goal, and each is expected to be accomplished within a designated time period. Sample objectives of caregiving and companion care are to:

refer care recipients to needed services and professionals
offer recreational activities during visits
examine home maintenance concerns on a regular basis
accomplish regularly scheduled errands to the grocery store, pharmacy, or other necessity

3.1

Exhibit

SMART (a widely used method for setting productive objectives).
S: specific, well defined
M: measurable (using numbers or comparisons)
A: attainable or achievable
R: realistic
T: timeline (defined time period)

These sample objectives meet the companion's overall goal to maintain and improve the quality of life for the care recipient while encouraging his or her independence for as long as possible. Objectives can be understood as action steps or a plan of care to achieve desired outcomes, and therefore, to achieve the goal(s) (see Exhibit 3.1). In caregiving situations, working with another or others is inevitable. It is more productive if everyone is following the same action steps to achieve the ultimate goal of quality client care.

Working With Others

Even working in a submarine on the ocean floor requires working with other people. Across industry lines, coworkers and teams work toward the same goal; being a companion home care provider is no different. Other employees may have different tasks and objectives, though the common purpose of home and home health care is to meet client needs. Teamwork is the two-way sharing of ideas and information with the anticipated outcome of helping each other. Effective teams successfully solve problems with creativity and efficiency. Characteristics of productive team members are communication, collaboration, approachability, and helpfulness. Team members can offer tips, techniques, and advice for handling complicated situations and managing tricky behaviors. They can also offer support and a listening ear or a shoulder to lean on during difficult times.

Case Study

Louise, in late stages of Alzheimer's, lived with her husband in their home. Doreen, Janice, and Kim provided companion care to Louise 7 days a week between 9:00 a.m. and 11:00 p.m.: Janice worked the Monday through Friday day shift, Doreen worked the evening shift Monday through Friday, and Kim was the daytime weekend companion. Janice and Doreen rotated the weekend night shift.

Janice was a single parent of four and frequently needed weekday hours for appointments. The three companion care providers decided that they would handle all scheduling conflicts and arrange for coverage with one another to not burden the already overwhelmed husband. They would switch shifts as able to accommodate last-minute changes. This was one less detail the husband had to tend to, and he was relieved that the care providers worked together to coordinate schedules and shift changes for coverage.

The care providers communicated mostly by telephone, though they did see each other at "shift change." Those few minutes were particularly helpful because Kim was new to working with Louise. Doreen and Janice had worked with Louise for 2 years and were able to provide Kim with practical tips and techniques for managing Louise's problem behaviors. They offered suggestions on how to get Louise to eat and ideas for spending recreational time. Doreen and Janice offered strategies for encouraging Louise up and down the stairs, which could take as long as 15 minutes to accomplish. Their combined information provided Kim with insight into the couple's preferences—likes and dislikes—that shortened her learning curve of their daily routines.

First and foremost, the client is the provider's teammate. A care provider works in the home with the client, usually alone, and may feel that they are the only person providing assistance, which is sometimes the case. More often than not there is someone else involved: family member, relative, friend, or neighbor. They are part of the team, especially if these informal caregivers provide aid or arrange for home care services. If possible, make connections with informal caregivers by introducing yourself, either by phone or face to face. Explain your role and how you will be aiding the care recipient. Clarify the services you will be providing and when you will be present. Initial and ongoing contact with this team can benefit the care recipient. Formal and informal caregivers who communicate regularly will be able to accommodate scheduling needs to ensure continued health and safety monitoring.

Case Study

Bonnie, 76 years old, was an only child and never married. She lived in the same home in which her parents raised her, continuing to live there over 50 years. She knew her immediate neighbors, a handful who had lived there 20 years. Bonnie was independent with decision making and was very active, mentally and socially. Since the progression of a nerve disorder she was limited to a wheelchair, but had enough mobility to transfer to her bed, couch, and toilet. As her physical condition deteriorated, Bonnie enlisted the help of her neighbors: Jenny walked Bonnie's dog every afternoon, Bob shoveled her driveway and brought in the trash cans, and Sally regularly picked up special food orders. Bonnie hired in other services, such as a housecleaner and pet-waste removal service; Holly did the grocery shopping and other errands. On occasion, Bonnie's stockbroker took her to inspect assisted living facilities.

Friends, neighbors, service personnel, and professionals were members of Bonnie's team. Each person completed needed tasks, contributing to her comfort, safety, and general well-being. This teamwork made it possible for Bonnie to stay living independently in her home.

Family members are teammates, though in various capacities. A companion must determine, through discussion or observation, (a) which family members want to be involved, (b) to what extent family members want to be involved, and (c) the frequency of contact those family members want with the companion caregiver. They should ask the family: Do they want to know what foods were purchased at the grocery store? The amount of the shopping bill? What prescriptions were filled and how much they cost? Inappropriate behaviors and incontinence issues? A full report from the doctor's visit, including written records from the doctor?

After family members define how they want to be involved, arrangements for continuing correspondence should be outlined. Is the care recipient able to accurately express wants and needs to the family or will the care provider communicate concerns and circumstances directly to the family through telephone calls, e-mails, or other forms of communication? The care provider should use documentation forms too, such as Figure 3.1. Which family member should receive a copy? Which family member needs phone calls for urgent matters? They should try to establish only one family member as a contact person to minimize confusion and to eliminate the need for repetitive telephone calls. If the companion or care provider works for an agency, there may be other staff who should be notified of emergencies and urgent matters, such as the nurse, social worker, or other home care provider. It is important to inform these team members when relaying care recipient needs and information because they may offer key links to essential resources or referrals. Input from the direct care provider helps professionals in these positions to coordinate appropriate services, therefore improving the care offerings and provisions to care recipients.

Emotions of Caring for Others

Caregiving situations can become overwhelming, stressful, and seemingly unmanageable. This is commonly known as "caregiver burnout." We typically think of family caregivers becoming exhausted with the responsibility of caring for another, though professional, formal caregivers can burn out from the responsibility of providing ongoing emotional support and attention.

Formal caregivers do not usually experience the same feelings of guilt or embarrassment that family caregivers can. These and other emotions may be felt, but for different reasons than the family caregivers. A formal care provider may experience guilt, but not because he or she made the decision to place the care recipient in a nursing home. The formal care provider may feel guilty for not being a stronger advocate for the care recipient or because the care provider revealed information about the care recipient that forced the family to make a decision for alternative living. Or, the caring companion thought he or she could do more to keep the care recipient living independently longer. It is the care provider's responsibility to determine if guilty feelings in such circumstances are rational or not.

A family or informal caregiver may experience anger because the care recipient does not perceive situations with good judgment, possibly jeopardizing their safety. The care provider may experience anger or frustration because the care recipient is unable to perform tasks as arranged or does not follow through with scheduled visits. As a companion, Jamie was scheduled to meet with Eleanor three times a week. Routinely and at the last minute, Eleanor would cancel one of those weekly visits. This not only left a void in Jamie's schedule, but Jamie could not complete tasks for Eleanor that required time constraints.

Feelings of isolation can be experienced by family and informal caregivers as well as formal caregivers. Home care providers spend typical days traveling from client to client and little time is spent with peers. They can feel cut off from the social networks of a workplace setting when the focus is on a care recipient's daily situations and routines.

Formal and informal caregivers will feel sadness when the care recipient or family member mentally or physically declines, and those who have established relationships with care recipients will experience grief during the dying process and when the care recipient does pass away. Laughter and love are also experienced in caregiving situations. Intimacy can develop and grow when caring for another person; a close, personal relationship with mutual understanding is very rewarding. As a companion to Rose, a care recipient with Alzheimer's disease, Robin felt overwhelmed with the sense of being needed every time Rose told Robin she loved her and asked, "Are you going to help me?" It is common for care recipients to regularly express appreciation to the care provider and may say such things as, "I do not know where I would be if you were not here to help" and "Thank you for taking care of me."

Other positive experiences in caregiving situations are a sense of satisfaction when a care provider is fulfilled by making a difference in another's life, and a sense of accomplishment when the care provider's service contributes to the comfort and safety of the care recipient.

Caregiver Burnout

What does it mean to *burn out?* It is best understood as a caregiver no longer finding fulfillment in his or her role, and the tasks of caregiving becoming unpleasant or even burdensome. How do professional care providers know when they are starting to burn out? Strong indicators of burnout are when the care provider becomes bored, uninterested, and easily irritated. As a result, it becomes difficult to communicate effectively and build close relationships with care recipients; therefore, service delivery suffers. Feeling overwhelmed with the general state of affairs and losing the ability to focus on care recipient needs are other warnings of burnout.

Repeatedly, professionals tell family caregivers that the best way to minimize stressors, manage challenging situations, and prevent burnout is to establish healthy boundaries. This same advice applies to formal care providers. What are healthy boundaries and how do they apply to professional care providers? Is setting healthy boundaries an effective or appropriate approach when working with confused care recipients?

To understand personal boundaries of the self and others is to understand that there are behavioral expectations and restrictions of what will and will not be tolerated. Individuals establish limits to what they find acceptable behavior (in personal life and in the workplace) before circumstances interfere with healthy mental and emotional functioning. This is a form of self-protection—a way to take care of the self and assume personal responsibility. Very simply, boundaries define what an individual is willing to accept to prevent relationship conditions from becoming problematic.

In the best-case scenario, setting boundaries looks like this:

Mary tells Mark her expectations and what behaviors are acceptable to her and why: *"Mark, it is not acceptable for you to be 15 minutes late for work every day because we have to wait for you to hold our morning meeting."*

Mary makes clear what action she will take to protect herself when Mark is late: *"Mark, I will have to take disciplinary action against you and keep a record of your tardiness in your file."*

Mary further details her action steps for protecting her boundary: *"If you continue to be late even after disciplinary action, I will have to terminate your employment."*

Stating personal boundaries should not be used as a method for manipulating or controlling other people to achieve personal outcomes. Clearly stated boundaries create and nurture healthy relationships. Setting boundaries requires honesty and direct communication. For successful relationships through boundary setting, another person must be willing to comply with the stated needs and expectations of tolerated behaviors. So, how can we expect a person with Alzheimer's, dementia, or other cognitive impairment to understand or remember our expressed boundaries? Is this an appropriate expectation from professionals specifically trained to work with cognitively impaired, lower functioning care recipients? Not really. In these exclusive situations, it is self-serving to state personal boundaries. If the care recipient needs assistance because of impaired cognition, why should they be expected to comprehend and meet our personal needs? Every person should continue to have limits and expectations of appropriate behaviors, but these need to be flexible in such unique circumstances. Care providers may be exposed to unpleasant and inappropriate conduct because of symptoms related to a client's deteriorating condition. If a care provider does not want to be subjected to clients who may use bad language or throw food because they lack cognition for social appropriateness, then this may not be a suitable job position.

A care provider needs to be compassionate and not lose patience when the care recipient cannot mentally comprehend directions to perform physical routines. The companion must have realistic expectations of what the care recipient is capable of managing and allow him or her the self-determination toward any effort of independence. Unrealistic expectations will produce feelings of anger, resentment, and frustration against the other person, creating stressful working relationships and conditions. The care provider should also be aware of his or her own competence (skills and talents) as well as personal tolerance levels to not assume responsibility for the care recipient, which creates dependency and unhealthy relationships (see Tip 3.3).

Tip 3.3

Quality Traits of a Companion and Home Care Provider

Energetic, creative, and flexible
Able to converse freely with different types of people
Motivates clients to act independently
Allows clients to feel useful and needed
Aware of personal boundaries and limitations
Able to communicate effectively
Compassionate and honest
Able to quickly establish rapport and build relationships
Ability to manage unpleasant tasks and difficult conversation topics
Able to manage frustration
Solution-focused to solve problems
Able to work with others
Educated about care options to offer clients and family

Self Care

Relieving Stress

There is ample scientific research on how stress impacts our emotional and physical well-being. Stress has been linked to: anxiety, fatigue, depression, sleep disorders, high blood pressure, heart attacks, and stomach and digestion problems. Stressful situations often occur between people as a result of a general lack of communication due to a misunderstanding of incomplete or inaccurate information. There is no way to completely avoid or eliminate stress. It is more effective to develop coping skills to manage situations of conflict that produce pressure and tension. The ability to be flexible, adjust to changing circumstances, and know what you can and cannot change contributes to stress reduction.

In addition to mental and emotional efforts that reduce stress, activity, and productivity have multiple benefits. Suggestions for recreational and stress-reducing activities can include:

Exercise (i.e., walking, jogging, yoga, bike riding, dancing, bowling)
Gardening
Meditation
Keeping a journal
Taking a bath

Reading
Shopping
Listening to relaxing music
Watching a movie
Sewing, knitting, quilting, crocheting, cross-stitching
Artwork (painting, drawing)
Spending time with friends and family

Personalizing Activities

Adding creativity to these relaxation techniques, Patty personalized her experiences as a home care provider by turning her workplace experiences into recreational and therapeutic hobbies.

Every week, Patty took two friends with Alzheimer's out to lunch followed by some type of recreational outing, such as to the art museum and special exhibits. She cut clippings from the newspaper or magazines that were relevant to their activities and collected brochures from each place visited. As a craft activity, Patty and the two clients covered scrapbook pages with decorative papers and affixed keepsakes. They glued on ribbons, buttons, and other accoutrements to make the book ornamental. They used the scrapbook during other visits to reminisce about familiar places and their outings.

Inspired by these same outings, Patty wrote short, simple stories that she used as activities with other clients. Patty read the stories to clients with advanced Alzheimer's disease who were able to understand the simple content and colorful descriptions. The simple stories served as pleasant remembrances of outings through age-appropriate reading material.

Gardening is one of Rhonda's pastimes, a hobby she shared with several of her clients. Rhonda helped some clients with plantings and gardening. As points of conversation throughout visits, Rhonda encourages discussion about favorite plants, flowers, and garden vegetables.

Dottie, one particular client with beginning Alzheimer's who lived in her own home, thoroughly enjoyed looking at flowers. Her family made sure that Dottie regularly had seasonal flowers in the home and yard. Rhonda spent over a year with Dottie before the family decided to move her to Colorado to live with her daughter. They had spent 5 days a week together; Rhonda was certain to miss Dottie. Rhonda planted a violet mum in her garden to be reminded of Dottie every August when it bloomed. Rhonda thought back on conversations with other clients about their favored flowers and planted one of each of those in her garden. The following March, Rhonda began visiting Mattie, who lived in a nursing home. Mattie became very special to Rhonda though she died within a month of their meeting. The family gathered friends at Mattie's house after the funeral and encouraged guests to take some of their mother's possessions, including garden flowers. The offering seemed fitting considering Rhonda's project, so she dug up Mattie's purple and white crocuses. Every spring, garden flowers remind Rhonda of Mattie. Rhonda thinks of another friend when the zinnias bloom and yet another client when the columbines blossom. Rhonda is growing her own memory garden!

There are many activities that promote relaxation. Every person has a unique style and expression for coping with stress. Essentially, any activity that pampers the self is recommended for minimizing stress. Different sources of stress may require different means for coping. Physical exertion releases tension that a restful activity, such as sewing, will not accomplish, and vice versa. Be creative when discovering your personal outlets.

Personal and Professional Growth

To learn is to grow, to grow is to learn. People learn from other people. We learn through books and classes. We learn by trying and doing, through hands-on experiences in the workplace and in personal life situations. Throughout our lifetimes, we accumulate information and knowledge that is used to form opinions and guide us when making decisions. Learning is more than data and information. It is applying the knowledge from the data and information for better problem solving and decision making, which makes good judgment possible. Thus, wisdom is born. Learning experiences expand our outlook and deepen our understanding. The more we learn and gain insight, the more we grow.

There is a large market of books, products, and peer-support systems dedicated to the personal growth market, also known as the self-help or self-improvement movement. The subject material focuses on motivation, inspiration, and stress management through the development of interpersonal skills. These practical skills are needed in the workplace and there is widespread interest in promoting professional as well as personal growth. The approaches to personal and professional growth are similar, though it appears that growing professionally entails assuming more responsibility and more challenging workplace projects to prove competencies. Typically, the desired outcome of professional growth is job satisfaction, career advancement, and financial benefits. Metaphorically, this translates in private life as personal satisfaction, accomplishment, incentive, and rewards.

An easy way of starting on a path toward self-improvement is creating personal mission and vision statements. Large posters stating an organization's mission and vision statements or principles of practice in how they interpret and provide quality care are often seen in home health care agencies, nursing homes, assisted living facilities, and other businesses. Personal mission and vision statements serve the same purpose for individuals. A personal vision statement is just that: the vision of your desired life. The personal mission statement describes the person's sense of meaning and purpose. It should be inspiring and unique to the person who creates the statement and does not have to be shared with others.

It is relevant to briefly mention the concept of Emotional Intelligence (EI) under the subject of personal and professional growth. The American Heritage Dictionary (2005) defines _emotional intelligence_ as "intelligence regarding the emotions, especially in the ability to monitor one's own or others' emotions." The term became popular in 1995 when Daniel Goleman wrote the book _Emotional Intelligence_ and several articles on the subject.

Cary Cherniss, PhD, presented "Emotional Intelligence: What It Is and Why It Matters" at the Annual Meeting of the Society for Industrial and Organizational Psychology in New Orleans, Louisiana, on April 15, 2000. Cherniss's focus is on the effectiveness of Emotional Intelligence (EI) in the workplace and how it improves efficiency and job satisfaction. According to Cherniss, Emotional Intelligence is the skill and talent of managing feelings, and knowing how and when to express them (Cherniss, 2000). This authentic self-control promotes productivity through the ability to manage stress while working with others. In the health care field, there is little way to avoid working with others. Obviously, the nature of being a care provider is to work one on one with others. This intimate work time presents plenty of opportunities for conflict and disagreements, which can be minimized with efforts to understand the other person. The more a person is able to identify, acknowledge, and manage his or her own feelings, the more capable he or she will be in perceiving and accepting others' thoughts and feelings. This is empathy, a result of adept Emotional Intelligence.

Controversy surrounds the subject; researchers disagree over the ability to measure an individual's Emotional Intelligence and if EI is intuitive abilities, cognitive skills, or a combination of both. Researchers are conducting studies on the role and value of Emotional Intelligence in conflict resolution and negotiation processes and how EI improves personal and professional relationships.

How does personal growth relate to caregiving and why is it important to a companion or other home care provider? Caregiving can be a demanding job with limited financial rewards; self-satisfaction can maximize the rewards of caregiving. A care provider who attempts to understand his or her own thoughts and emotions can gain insight into the unspoken thoughts and feelings of the care recipient. The ability to perceive another person's hidden nature is useful for understanding what motivates that person to action or even inaction. This becomes an important part of providing care, especially to care recipients who are unable to clearly express desires and needs. Empathy is an essential attribute of a quality care provider.

Summary

A companion is an integral member of the formal or informal caregiving system, providing communication links and supervision to the client. Companions offer assistance with Instrumental Activities of Daily Living (IADLs) for managing routine household functions; Activities of Daily Living (ADLs) entail personal care routines and should be performed by trained professionals. The companion's goal is to keep the client safe with the best quality of life offerings possible in the living environment of choice.

Teamwork is an integral element of caring for others. The client is the care provider's number one teammate but in most situations there are others involved, such as family members, friends, health care providers, and other professionals. Care providers should develop healthy relationship-building skills by knowing personal limits and not forcing unrealistic expectations on clients, which can be accomplished by understanding clients' abilities and limitations. Unrealistic expectations produce feelings of anger, resentment, and frustration, creating difficult working relationships. The ability to manage stress helps a person maximize energy to focus on issues of meaning, which improves work and personal relationships. Personal and professional growth, and eventually to self-awareness and satisfaction is developed through the learning process. Personal mission and vision statements are guidelines toward self-improvement. The statements are reflections of thought on the positive qualities an individual desires to attain.

Emotional Intelligence is the awareness and management of personal emotions and needs while understanding the emotions and needs of another person. A strong sense of Emotional Intelligence contributes to efficient problem solving and conflict resolution. The end results of monitoring individual emotions and responses are the ability to manage stress, increase productivity, and improve working relationships with peers and care recipients.

Questions

What is the difference between ADLs and IADLs?
What are the roles and responsibilities of the companion care provider?
Why is documenting client behavior important?
What are the objectives and goals of a companion caregiver?
How can defining goals and objectives improve service delivery?
What are typical feelings experienced by formal and informal caregivers?
What does it mean to develop healthy relationships?
Think of a situation when you let your emotions get out of control. How could that situation have been managed differently?
How is personal and professional growth significant to care providers?

Summary Tips

Be clear on what goals and objectives need to be accomplished with each client.
Documenting client needs and behaviors after each visit creates an ongoing log to better monitor for changes in the client. It also sets up a system of communication with family or other caregivers.
Clearly state expectations and goals for better results: know your personal boundaries, limits, and expectations to improve relationships.
Discover personal relaxation techniques and practice them regularly.

Helpful Web Sites

ADLs and IADLs: http://www.answers.com/topic/activities-of-daily-living?cat=biz-fin
Emotional Intelligence: Institute for Health and Human Potential at http://www.ihhp.com/what_is_eq.htm
Medical terminology: http://www.medterms.com/script/main/hp.asp
Mission and vision statements: http:// www.missionvisionstatement.com

Suggested Reading

Benson, Herbert. (2000). *The relaxation response*. New York: HarperCollins. Simple and effective approaches for managing stress.
Buscaglia, Leo. (1985). *Living, loving, and learning*. New York: Random House. Insights on love, interpersonal relations, and self-actualization.

Carter, Rosalyn. (1995). *Helping yourself help others: A book for caregivers.* New York: Crown Publishing Group. A personal account of caregiving and practical solutions to problems often faced by caregivers.

Covey, Stephen R. (1999). *First things first.* New York: Simon and Schuster. An inspirational and practical approach to effective time-management skills and relationships.

Gawain, Shakti. (1998). *Creative visualization.* Novato, CA: New World Library. Easy and practical methods for using the power of imagination to change negative habits and improve self-esteem.

Siegel, Bernie. (1986). *Love, medicine, and miracles.* New York: HarperCollins. A doctor shares lessons learned from patients about their participation in self-healing and recovery.

Interpersonal Skills and Communications

4

In This Chapter, You Will Learn

1. Personal skills of a care provider

2. To identify communication skills:

   Conversation
   Listening
   Problem solving
   Conflict resolution
   Decision making

3. To identify family roles and dynamics

4. Observation skills using the five senses

Why This Matters

Interacting with others occurs daily for most people. We discuss schedules and social events with our spouses, parents, and children. We gossip and talk about tasks with coworkers. We ask friends for advice and store associates for assistance. We share ideas, plan social events, solve problems, help others, and make decisions while conversing with others. How we exchange verbal and nonverbal information creates successful communications. What skills could you improve to communicate more effectively? Positive communications improve personal and working relationships, efficiency, and productivity. Home care providers meet many people and personality types. A broad set of communication skills are needed to communicate effectively with coworkers, care recipients, and family members. This chapter offers suggestions to strengthen skills for successful, positive communications. It takes time to communicate better; with improved relationships and personal satisfaction as results, it is worth the effort.

Personal Skills

Caregiving requires a special skill set, personality and temperament that not every person has. A care recipient is in some type of compromised situation by the time a care provider enters the scene, which is why such services are arranged. The needs of each care recipient will be different and every caregiving situation is unique, which means that care providers must adapt to changing circumstances and dynamics. Care providers should possess three essential characteristics: patience, understanding, and compassion.

Patience means being flexible with varying dynamics, such as changes in schedules, routines, and responses. Flexibility is important when dealing with personalities and just as important when managing schedules. Reasons why a care provider's work schedule can change unexpectedly may be due to sudden health emergencies, urgent appointments, cancelled appointments, or the care recipient just not feeling well enough for the care provider's visit. The care provider should be tolerant and understanding of last-minute schedule changes when a care recipient is unable to provide much prior notice.

Every person processes thoughts, ideas, and feelings in a different manner. Care providers should attempt to understand each care recipient's style and approach. Few people complete a given task in the same manner. The care recipient has been performing practices and applying techniques for many years. There is no reason that habits should change at this later and potentially more challenging time of life. Learning about a care recipient's background and history may provide insight into a care recipient's conduct. The care provider should ask about the care recipient's life during childhood and adulthood, and throughout conversations inquire about likes and dislikes to learn more about the care recipient's personality. If appropriate, they can talk about the care recipient's current condition and offer support. A care provider who is friendly, outgoing, and conversant will form faster rapport and friendships.

Care providers should act with compassion to current circumstances. Encouraging and motivating a care recipient as a means to promote independence is supportive, but expecting that the care recipient can accomplish tasks they were previously able to complete may be impractical. Be thoughtful of life changes that are currently happening or have occurred for the care recipient and put yourself in the position of a care recipient: It cannot be easy to rely on others for daily tasks and care that were once accomplished independently.

Communication Skills

In addition to personality traits, communication skills (also called interpersonal skills) are necessary for establishing personal connections and building relationships with care recipients, family members, and other professionals. Successful communication is paramount when working with people. Personal bonds are not created and relationships are not formed without proper communication or understanding. Communication is simply the exchange of information through verbal (speech) or nonverbal (writing, signals, and expressions) means. The difficulty in communicating is how needs, thoughts, and feelings are expressed to others. The first consideration is which mode of communication to use to send the message, then to choose appropriate and accurate words or messages to effectively convey meaning.

Quality communication skills are indispensable that result in resourceful, fruitful, and cooperative outcomes. Conversation, listening, problem solving, conflict resolution, and decision making are interpersonal skills to develop for effective communication (see Figure 4.1). These factors are the basics of how

4.1

Components of effective communication

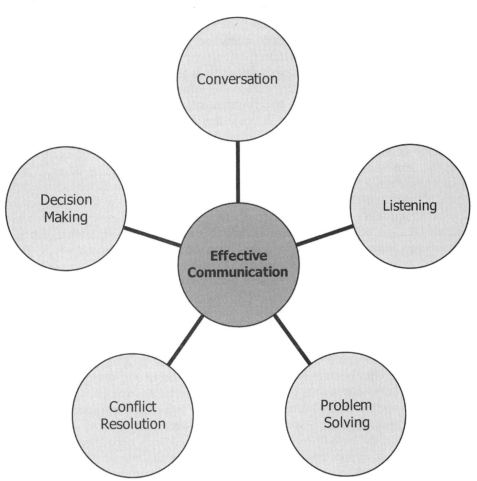

we communicate with others. Our abilities in these skill areas reflect how we relate and interact with others. Communication skills develop over time with effort and experience. The following suggestions can directly improve interactions and relationships:

Understand your perspective
Look at situations from another's point of view to understand their perspective
Pay attention to nonverbal cues: facial expressions, eye contact, posture, body movements, and gestures
Pay attention to verbal cues: volume, tone, and word choice
Use active listening: focus on speaker, do not think about what you'll say next, and ask related questions
Ask open-ended questions to encourage a speaker to elaborate on wants and needs, thoughts and opinions
Ask for feedback and advice
Know when not saying anything is best

Most people care more that they are heard and listened to than whether the listener agrees with their thoughts or opinions. A care provider is often in the position of being that listener. In many caregiving situations, care recipients want an objective listener to whom they can express feelings and fears regarding current or future circumstances rather than advice on what he or she should or should not do. Care recipients tend to feel vulnerable when sharing thoughts and feelings with their family and physician for fear of how these others will respond and react to the shared information. A concern often heard from care recipients is that if they give certain others too much information about the areas for needed assistance, their decision-making rights will be taken away and the care recipient will be subject to the decisions made by others. Often, a care recipient's perception is that sharing with a care provider is less risky toward unwanted change. The care provider does not need to have answers as the care recipient processes actual or anticipated challenges; answers are less important than offering the care recipient attentive listening. Other times, a care recipient finds comfort just in sharing meaningful stories and events from the past, otherwise known as reminiscing. When the relationship between a care provider and care recipient is well established, the care recipient may seek further input from the care provider. In this case, the care provider can treat the conversation and the care recipient with respect by asking questions and contributing comments.

It is especially important to watch body language and facial expressions of nonverbal care recipients to determine personal needs. When working with a care recipient who is unable to verbalize wants and needs, the best communications are simple questions that require a yes or no answer. If physically able, encourage the care recipient to write messages and communications. The nonverbal care recipient can respond with head movements if he or she is physically and cognitively able to comprehend. People with advanced Alzheimer's disease or other dementia can lose the ability to articulate or speak and communications can be challenging. A care recipient who cannot verbalize possibly does not comprehend the content of conversations or the questions being asked.

Care providers must rely on their intuition and judgment, and their ability to ask pertinent questions with an understandable approach, to determine the needs of the care recipient. In these situations, it is strongly suggested to continue talking to the care recipient because it provides stimulation and human contact, which can calm the care recipient or de-escalate tense dynamics. It appears to help the care recipient feel connected, which also helps strengthen the unspoken bonds between care provider and care recipient.

Care providers can develop quality communications by improving conversation and listening skills as well as problem-solving, conflict-resolution, and decision-making abilities. Many times the care provider may need to make in-the-moment suggestions and judgments, especially when alone with the care recipient. Expanding these communication skills for personal and professional growth takes time, understanding, and practice.

Communicating With Family

Every family has a unique code of communication for sharing and processing information; within the family system, each member has perceptions and experiences that affect how information and events are individually interpreted. The variances of responses and reactions among family members can cause tension or conflict, which may prohibit cooperative planning and decision making; of importance is how family communications are impacting the current caregiving situation. Family members' perceived roles can present serious challenges in caregiving situations particularly when family members disagree over the direction of care a parent should receive. To work together toward quality care, it is best for a care provider to suspend judgment: It is likely that the care provider is hearing one side of the story from a family member and is lacking perspective from others. Other sources of family conflict are:

A history of poor communicating and relationship difficulties
Varying perspectives that prohibit cooperative decision making
Family secrets or situational stories that some members want kept private
Feelings of guilt or anger at the parent or other family members
One family member assuming more responsibility (time, assistance, money) than others
Unequal decision-making capacities, such as when one person dictates what will happen with the client (usually, the parent) and does not include other family members in the decision-making process
Lack of resources, such as time, money, and people

Caring for a loved one usually adds stress on families who are already strained because of the past or present shifting roles of family members including care recipients, especially when a health matter requires urgent decisions. End-of-life decision making, such as withholding or withdrawing measures of life support, can lead to extremely difficult emotional circumstances. Another dilemma occurs when the care recipient is considered independent with decision making though lacking in good judgment. Family members want to balance the care recipient's need for independent decision making with the need for safety and well-being. Furthermore, there will be caregiving dynamics created by family members who want to control the circumstances by setting unrealistic expectations and imposing decisions on the family member receiving care, who is still independent with decision-making capabilities.

Care recipients or family members may provoke situations and act in a manipulative manner. These situations usually occur because there is a need that is not being met and the care recipient or family members become desperate. The best approach a home care provider can take during these unpleasant situations is to listen to the other person, identify what the need is, and follow steps for problem solving or conflict resolution to act in the best interest for the care recipient.

The home care provider should advocate for care recipients' best interests by focusing on their needs, being careful not to get in the middle of family feuding. It is not the care provider's responsibility to resolve family conflicts. Some people are more receptive to the suggestion of seeking outside support when this advice comes from a nonfamily member. Care providers can recommend that family members attend support groups or talk with a social worker if relationships are seriously strained. It may be necessary to advise that one or all family members talk with a professional counselor.

Conversation Skills

Conversation is a form of art that takes effort and practice. It is more than the standard greetings that are offered out of politeness to strangers and acquaintances that we pass on the street. A conversation is a meaningful exchange between two or more people about beliefs, values, and feelings, whether expressed verbally or through another mode of communication such as writing messages, facial gestures, and body movements.

How does a person practice improving conversations to become a better conversationalist?

Focus on the other person. Truly listen to what is being said. One way to put this into practice is committing yourself to ask the other person at least one question relevant to the topic of discussion. If too many questions are asked, the person speaking may think the message is not being clearly conveyed.

Learn the other person's interests. Be interested; there is always time to learn more. If you do not know the subject matter, ask questions. Or, find a topic that you are familiar with and make comparisons. For example, if the person is talking about the art museum and you have never been, relate your experience from another museum.

Listen attentively. Questions and comments are a good way to convey that you are listening. When used appropriately, not responding and allowing the speaker time to express him- or herself shows attentive listening. Nonverbal signs (eye contact and appropriate head nods) that demonstrate listening are also important. One word replies (yes, no, ok, sure) also validate what is being said.

Use active listening skills. Offer your opinions, being careful not to sound judgmental or critical. Words and phrases to say could be "I see," "That makes sense," or "I do not understand," which all acknowledge the speaker's comments.

Stick to "safe" conversations. If you are a care provider for an older adult, there are likely differences in social attitudes, perceptions, and values. Be prepared to hear how current times are different from the care recipient's younger years and avoid controversial subjects that could potentially lead to disagreements.

These suggestions contribute to the process of becoming a better conversationalist, but how does one get started? Knowledge of various topics is always helpful, though working your way into unfamiliar subjects can be done by asking questions and comparing your experiences to the points of conversation. The newspaper, or other news supply, is a good source for keeping up with current events. Some care recipients, particularly those with Alzheimer's disease or dementia, may not be able to keep up with current events nor is the content relevant to their circumstances. Small talk about the weather, a football game, last night's dinner, or a story from the news are fine conversation starters. These polite conversations may set the tone as "this care provider is easy to talk with" for the care recipient, who may feel safe with communicating and openly sharing their viewpoints. This type of conversation can be a pleasant distraction from a care recipient's current conditions, or for the care recipient who is guarded with their personal matters and information.

Other suggestions for starting conversations are to discuss

An event from your daily, weekly, or monthly routines
Care provider and care recipient hobbies
Favorite restaurants, delis, and bakeries
Favorite recipes, desserts, and other foods
Childhood or adult heroes and idols
Favorite movies, actors and actresses, books, authors, and characters
Neighborhoods that the care provider or care recipient lived in during childhood and adulthood
What care provider or care recipient does with weekend, vacation, and recreational time
The care recipient's occupation (to add intrigue—if they could have any job in the world, what would it be?)

Tips for Communicating With Older Adults

Cognitive or sensory impairments can impact communications with some care recipients. The following suggestions are particularly helpful when working with the older adult population:

Speak slowly and clearly
Allow the person time to respond
Speak to the person as an adult
Use manners and be courteous
Address by name or lightly touch him or her to get their attention
Make eye contact when speaking
Eliminate noises and distractions when conversing
Use facial or physical gestures to help send messages

Avoid vague words, such as *it, this, that,* and *there*

Use nouns—call objects by correct name

Use titles, phrases, and descriptive words that are familiar to the person

Offer words when a person cannot recall without completing their thoughts and sentences

Avoid details with those who have difficulty remembering

Offer a few choices; do not overwhelm the person with options

Phrase questions and statements with positive words: rather than "Don't do that," ask, "Would you like to consider (fill in the blank) instead?"

Do not disagree; validate their feelings

Offer gentle reminders to calm a person

Look for feelings beyond words: persons affected by Alzheimer's, dementia, or stroke may not be able to recall or articulate appropriate words

Listening Skills

Listening is more than repeating words and thoughts back to the speaker. To listen is to identify the words that create a message, then to process that message into understanding the speaker's needs, values, thoughts, and feelings. A good listener watches and listens to the speaker for a consistent message to offer feedback through questions, comments, opinions, or suggestions.

Knowingly or not, people communicate unmet needs and express themselves with the expectation that a want or need will be recognized, even if the need is simply to be heard. A good listener tries sincerely to appreciate the speaker's wants and needs, and how he or she thinks and feels.

Distraction with other thoughts creates a barrier to becoming an effective listener. How often have you found yourself thinking about errands or grocery lists or planning social activities when someone is trying to tell you something? Replying with prepared phrases and clichés for what should follow next in a conversation creates barriers to effective listening. Intentionally or not, we may have a response prepared to defend ourselves—"This wasn't my fault," or "I didn't do it," or "The important thing is …"—rather than hearing what is being expressed. Another barrier to effective listening (and communicating) is judging what the speaker says, whether by thinking or actually saying, "That is a bad idea, it will never work." Instead, listen and hear what is being said and understand what need is not being met.

To become a better listener:

Focus on the speaker. Give your full attention to what the speaker is saying and ask yourself, "What is the main point this person is trying to make?" If your mind starts to wander, redirect your thoughts to the speaker and make an effort to find meaning in the message.

Make eye contact. This lets the speaker know that you are focusing on their words and messages and makes it easier for you to stay focused. Be aware of their body language as well as your own.

Try not to interrupt; let the speaker finish the sentence. Some care recipients, especially the elderly or others with chronic conditions, may be slower to respond or have difficulty finding the appropriate words to express their thoughts. Allow them time to respond and use judgment when completing a sentence for them. Providing words as gentle reminders to keep the care recipient focused is acceptable, but take caution not to misconstrue the other person's message with your own words and thoughts.

Ask questions. This will help to clarify the speaker's message to make sure you understand what is being asked or said. If what is being said is not understood, let the speaker know and ask him or her to explain the message again with a different approach. Asking good questions will improve conversation skills.

Give feedback. Put the speaker's words in your own and repeat it back to them to clarify your understanding of the message. There is no guarantee that a person is listening or understanding just because words are repeated. Restate the facts, wants, needs, thoughts, and feelings, and then make a suggestion on how to proceed if a plan of action is needed.

Use a nonjudgmental and empathetic approach. Assisting others is not about projecting your values and beliefs or telling them what to do; it is about being tolerant and respectful of another person's perceptions.

Attentive Listening

After a fall that resulted in a broken hip, Carolyn moved into assisted living. Her daughter lived out of town and hired Anita to visit three times a week to make sure that Carolyn had what she wanted and needed as she adjusted to life in a facility. Carolyn regularly talked about the past and her husband's work as a successful business owner of a factory on the south side of town. During the time Anita provided service to her, a factory on the city's south side shut down operations. Anita told Carolyn about the factory's closing, hoping the news could be relevant and would spark some interest. As it turned out, she was very familiar with the factory: Her husband had owned that same factory over 40 years ago!

The current news event was a successful conversation starter because Anita made an effort to connect with Carolyn from Carolyn's point of view. During Anita's time with Carolyn, she listened to—not just heard—Carolyn's stories to gain understanding of what was of interest to her and what subjects would be related to her past experiences and personal connections. Anita was not only able to share information with her, but she also validated Carolyn's need to be heard through the listening process: Anita heard her words and messages and was able to offer insightful feedback that demonstrated to Carolyn that Anita had been listening attentively.

There are unintentional causes that obstruct effective listening. Because the care recipient who is being assisted has somewhat compromised functioning— or else there would be no need for the care provider's service—there may be communication difficulties beyond the care recipient's control.

Alzheimer's disease, dementia, CVA (Cerebrovascular disease, known as stroke), or other degenerative brain conditions can affect how a person relays information. The care recipient may speak softly or sentences may be incomplete, making it difficult for a listener to hear and comprehend what is being said. As the result of a disease, the care recipient may not have appropriate words to accurately express wants and needs. Long phrases and descriptive words may be used instead of one-word or shorter explanations to communicate a thought or concept. This requires conscientious listening, in which the listener must visualize what is being said to then put into their own context. Strokes and certain dementias can affect speech patterns in this way, where the person is unable to recall nouns and will readily use adjectives or other filler words to describe the idea.

Listening skills are a building block of the communication process. To practice effective listening, acknowledge what the other person is saying by reflecting the message back to the person: "That sounds like an exciting experience!" or "You sound very upset by what the doctor has told you," or "I'm sorry you have to think about moving from your home." Restate, in your own words, what the person has said to demonstrate understanding; for example, "Are you saying that you are going to look for other living arrangements?" or "It sounds that if you do not get the home services you need, you may have to find an alternative living situation." Check your understanding by asking open-ended questions: "What type of home services do you need?" or "What other services can be arranged to help you live independently longer?"

There will be care recipients who will not share their opinions and feelings, especially to family members, because they fear that family members will make decisions against their wishes or because it will add burden to an already stressful situation. There will be care recipients who are private with their personal matters and do not want to share how they truly feel. It is important to be considerate of the care recipient's privacy and cautious in sharing sensitive information with others. Remember, the care recipient has physical, mental, and emotional needs that must be met. Communication patterns are as old as an individual; do not expect a change in these established habits. A care provider should listen and be aware of what a care recipient is and is not saying, giving attention to facial expressions, tone and volume of voice, posture, and gestures.

A care provider should continually practice listening skills to improve communications and build relationships. Many times, the care provider is the informational link between the care recipient, family, or other care providers. The care provider needs to clearly understand the care recipient's wants and needs in order to relay correct information. This will ensure that the care recipient is able to function independently, or as well as possible, in the living situation.

Problem-Solving Skills

The problem-solving process creates opportunities to achieve desired results. Problems are solved every day. Stop and think: What did you have to consider when making alternative arrangements to get to work because your car would not start? How did you cope when the presentation was in an hour and you realized the materials were at home? Knowingly or not, problem-solving skills were used to accomplish what needed to be done. Basic problem-solving skills are:

Analyzing the situation
Defining the problem

Brainstorming ideas
Researching options
Negotiating terms
Selecting the best option
Evaluating outcomes

Applying these skills is the problem-solving process (see Table 4.1, Steps Toward Better Problem Solving). Define the problem by using the five "Ws": what is the problem, why does it happen, who is involved, where is the break down, and when do the issues occur. Next, think about the options that may solve the problem, considering the advantages and disadvantages of each potential solution. What are potential consequences? Who will be impacted and how will their needs be affected? To determine the best solution, again use the five "Ws": why is it the best solution, what are the advantages and disadvantages, where will it take place, when will it take place, and who will be responsible for applying the plan. This stage takes planning and organization to ensure that all involved understand the plan of action for accomplishment. Before evaluating the results, allow time for the chosen option to be effective. Then, consider if the solution is working, why or why not, and how it could be improved.

In the event of more than one problem at a time, the problem solver must also exercise priority and judge which problem must be dealt with first. One way of determining priority in caregiving situations is to first evaluate the urgency for medical attention and safety concerns. A problem situation that threatens or puts the care recipient at physical risk should be top priority. If there is time to deal with the matter, follow the steps in Table 4.1. Do not forget about team members; ask for advice from peers and other professionals. If there is less time, create the legendary pro and con list. In emergencies, quickly review the steps and make the best possible decision in the limited amount of time. There is always the do-nothing approach, but this should be used carefully in caregiving situations. Doing nothing may be detrimental in urgent situations.

The care recipient's point of view should always be considered in problem-solving situations. If a care recipient is not consulted, it will appear that the care provider is making decisions for the care recipient. Certain circumstances may not make much difference to the care provider though it could be of great significance to the care recipient. Depending on the urgency of the matter, the brainstorming process may be more important than having an immediate answer. The care recipient may appreciate that the time is taken to work through a difficult situation, which will demonstrate that the care provider is ready and willing to work as a team.

Personality types influence the individual and group problem-solving process. There is too much information on personality and learning styles to examine here, though a vast amount of research about types of personalities, including online tests and tutorials to determine learning and personality types. These tests help identify preferences, attitudes, and behaviors toward solving problems. It is helpful for personal and professional growth to have a general idea of what your personality style is to understand how you will interpret and manage situations. In order to work cooperatively with others, it is also helpful

4.1 Steps Toward Better Problem Solving

Define problem and set goal	Explore options	Select best option	Evaluate
■ Examine situation	■ Brainstorm: think creatively and logically	■ Does the best option meet the needs?	■ Did the best option work?
■ Gather information			■ Why or why not?
■ What are the needs?	■ What are potential consequences?	■ Why is it the best option?	■ What were positive and negative impacts?
■ The 5 Ws:	■ What are the advantages and disadvantages?	■ What are the estimated advantages and disadvantages?	■ What are the found advantages and disadvantages?
1) *Who* is involved?	■ Do options meet the needs?	■ Who will put the action plan into practice?	■ Are there ways to improve the action plan?
2) *What* is the problem?	■ What is impact on	■ Who will regularly provide the course of action?	■ What is feedback from recipient? Others?
3) *Where* is the problem? (with a routine, system, or other involved person?)	*Provider?*		
4) *When* does the problem occur? (regularly or episodic?)	*Client?*	■ How will it get started?	
	Others?	■ Where will it take place?	
5) *Why* does it occur? (personality conflict, schedule conflict, or related to health or medical concerns?)		■ What will need to occur?	
		■ What is needed?	
		■ When will it start? End?	

to understand how other people perceive situations and circumstances. This requires looking at all facets of the situation from other points of view. The art and skill of working with people is the ability to know which approach to use and when to use it appropriately.

Conflict-Resolution Skills

Conflict happens when one person says or does something that results in another person feeling threatened that a personal need will not be met. The person who feels threatened experiences negative emotions and responds unconstructively to the initial behavior or threat. In turn, the person who—intentionally or not—initiated the threat will react negatively. The cycle of conflict begins and continues until one or both people make an effort to resolve the problem. Effective conflict resolution will result in a win-win situation with mutual benefits for both, which will also improve the relationship.

The concept and practice of conflict resolution implies two or more people working together to find a solution to a setback or a crisis. A safe environment to share needs, fears, and feelings is critical; usually, a third person who is a trained professional or specialist facilitates the resolution process, known as mediation or arbitration. The involved parties can work toward resolution together in less extreme situations. In most caregiving situations, the care provider and the care recipient will reach agreement, sometimes with the help of family members or other agency employees.

It helps to have an idea of how you manage situations of conflict. Understanding your approach to conflict resolution is an element of effective communication. Different styles of conflict resolution can be applied depending on the circumstances, situation, and nature of the relationship with the other involved. Awareness of personal position and perceptions gives insight into what should or should not be the focus of attention. This gap of information is where the most learning occurs: What is not given initial attention could be exactly the other person's point of view. Considering personal style and approach is also enlightening to how others think; you will begin to look at other people from this framework, which will help you understand situations from other points of view. Ultimately, this enhances communications and deepens relationships. Resolving conflicts becomes easier and more successful in the meantime.

How do people work together to resolve a conflict? For a problem to exist, the people involved must first recognize that there is a problem. There are at least two people concerned and the conflict needs to be addressed as a partnership to meet the needs of the individuals involved. This requires open sharing of how each person involved in the dispute views the circumstances; through this process, the problem is clarified. Together, involved parties can make suggestions and recommendations on how to solve the conflict. An action plan that establishes tasks and responsibilities can then be prepared. Everyone involved should be willing to agree that an effort will be put forth to settle the dispute. The action plan and verbal or written agreements should be evaluated frequently when the changes are first put into practice, and then monitored regularly to make sure the plans are working. See Table 4.2 for approaching conflict resolution.

4.2 Steps Toward Conflict Resolution

Identify and clarify the problem	• Involved parties understand each other's perceptions of the problem
	• Is the difference over:
	    Wants and needs?
	    Values and beliefs?
	    Approach?
	    End goal?
	• Identify problem behaviors
	• Clarify misstated or misunderstood facts

Determine needs of those involved	• Individual needs • Shared needs • Other priorities
Generate options	• Brainstorm ideas • Each person make suggestions for improving situation • Input from all involved as to why or why not the suggestion will or will not work
Create action plan	• Clarify who will do what • Set timelines as needed • Understand the goal or intended end result of each action step
Make agreements	• Agree to follow outlined action plan • Regularly evaluate if the plans are working

Depending on the nature of the conflict, the process of resolving conflicts can be similar to solving problems, though they address different issues. When brainstorming ideas to make a care recipient's home adaptable, problem-solving skills are used, because the conflict is not with other involved parties. Conflict resolution is the result of two (or more) people agreeing to work toward finding a common goal in the middle of disagreement.

Determine if the following scenarios use conflict-resolution or problem-solving skills:

A care recipient with osteoporosis has trouble reaching higher than her shoulder level to open kitchen cabinets. The care provider and recipient discuss various ideas, such as moving items from the upper cupboards into the lower cupboards, placing regularly used kitchen items on the counter, or tying long strings for easy grabbing on the upper cupboard door handles. The care recipient decides that tying strings on the door handles is the best decision because it enables her to open the cabinets and is the most trouble-free choice.

The care recipient has been resistant to assistance in the home but reluctantly agreed to the family's demand. The family has asked the care provider to arrive every Monday at 1:00 p.m. When the care provider shows up, the care recipient is frequently eating lunch; therefore, the care provider is unable to take the care recipient to the grocery store and run other errands that the family has requested. Due to finances, the care recipient has asked that the scheduled time not exceed 2 hours. After much deliberation, the care provider and the care recipient agree that later afternoon hours would be a better time to accomplish tasks for better service provisions.

A family has asked that the care provider report to them after each weekly visit with their slightly forgetful mother. This serves more than one purpose. The care provider is informing the family that he or she did indeed show up at the times scheduled and observations of mom's behaviors and cognitive functioning are relayed to the family; they are informed of the day's activities, including what foods were bought at the grocery store. On one trip to the grocery, the care recipient bought cinnamon rolls, frozen biscuits, ice cream, and diet cola. The care provider reported to the purchases to the daughter, not realizing that her mother is diabetic. The daughter scolded her mother, the care recipient, for not following her diabetic diet. The care recipient was upset with the care provider for sharing too much information with her daughter. The care recipient states that if the care provider continues to correspond with her daughter or other family members, she will terminate services.

The nature of working with others always presents the potential for conflict, whether in personal or professional situations. Being a care provider presents situations of conflict at varying degrees, over large and small circumstances. Formal and informal caregivers work with care recipients, their families and friends, health care professionals, and other professionals. All involved may have different perceptions and opinions of what type of care is needed and how care will be provided. When there can be input and direction from so many others, consensus for quality care must be reached. This is the goal to resolve disagreements, and strong conflict-resolution skills achieve this goal.

Decision-Making Skills

Everyone makes decisions every day. What did you decide to eat for breakfast? What outfit did you choose to wear? What attitude did you decide to have today? What decisions were made last week?

Decision making is the process of considering possible actions or thought choices and then choosing an option. As in the problem-solving process, the way we make decisions is influenced significantly by our personality and learning styles. Decisions are based on factual information, or on assumptions and intuition of how circumstances are felt and perceived. Decisions come with varying degrees of intensity; choosing what to wear generally has fewer implications than decisions that will affect a person's health or financial position. There are several considerations in any decision, especially those that impact a person's well-being. First, what are the options and alternatives? What are the benefits and risks of each option? What does each option involve and what are the expected outcomes? Finally, what is the expected result of the final decision?

Problem-solving models and methods are used to weigh the advantages and disadvantages of a given situation. The following guidelines offer a general approach:

Identify the decision that needs to be made
Brainstorm the advantages and disadvantages of possible options
Select an option
Implement an action plan
Evaluate the action plan, making changes as necessary

It is unlikely that home care providers will make life-altering decisions for care recipients, though care providers interpret and convey information to those who do make significant decisions. On a day-to-day basis, care providers' decisions may set the parameters and schedules of what should happen when working with the care recipient or family. Addressing details and exploring options before making a big decision, such as long-term-care placement, contributes to the success of the care recipient remaining independent for as long as possible.

Communications is a broad subject, and involves more than just improving interpersonal skills. People communicate because they have unmet needs and unfulfilled wants. The skills discussed—conversation, listening, problem solving, conflict resolution, and decision making—present a broad framework for enhancing communication.

Observation Skills

Interpersonal skills focus on expressed wants and needs, but what about the unstated wants and needs of the care recipient? For different reasons, a care recipient may not always be able to articulate, express, or verbalize wants and needs. Neurological conditions can affect cognitive functioning or speech, making proper articulation and verbalization difficult. A care recipient may choose not to share or verbalize wants and needs to protect privacy, or has never learned how to express the self appropriately. Care providers must use their ability to recognize nonverbal messages through general observations during visits. Observations can supply more insight into the care recipient's state of affairs and well-being than what is actually verbalized. Care providers can learn to accurately read care recipients' unspoken messages through their body language and nonverbal communications. Moods and thoughts may be expressed through eye contact, facial expressions, body gestures, posture, and habits. The care provider who develops acute observation skills can learn to identify what is not being verbalized and consider if what is being said is consistent with care needs and is reasonable for the situation. These observations can be used as a measuring stick for a change in the care recipient's functioning status. Regardless of how information is communicated, the care provider will gain insight into the care recipient by observing actions, attitudes, behaviors, and the living environment.

What words, actions, and behaviors are important to observe to determine what the care recipient may not be saying?

Appearance

Physical appearance and demeanor is a strong indicator of a person's energy level, motivation, and desire for good personal care. The physical presentation of a care recipient often reflects how he or she is feeling physically and emotionally. Care providers should be alert to the messages. Is the care recipient tidy or unkempt? Are the clothes clean? Does the care recipient appear over- or underdressed? If eyeglasses, dentures, or hearing aids are necessary, is the care recipient wearing them regularly? Personal hygiene habits are observable through physical appearance. Does hair look washed? Have teeth been brushed? Are fingernails broken and uneven? The care recipient's appearance can indicate a changing emotional or physical status that requires closer supervision. Is the shirt that is tucked in every day buttoned haphazardly today? Is the care recipient typically dressed and ready for the care provider's visit but has been in sleepwear for the past three visits? Has hair that is usually brushed nicely been uncombed for the last week?

Appearance is a strong indicator of the level of care a care recipient is receiving in an assisted living or long-term-care facility. If a care recipient continually looks unclean and is regularly wearing dirty clothes, it is a safe assumption that the care recipient is not being showered nor is laundry being cleaned. (Though before assuming that the staff is neglecting care, it is a good idea to find out why expected care routines are not being performed. Is the care recipient refusing care or is he or she having difficulty adjusting to the new living situation, and do other issues need to be addressed?)

Mood

Many times, a care recipient's mood is noticeable by the way he or she physically carries the body. A slumped posture and low shoulders could be a sign of tiredness or sadness. If this posture becomes a regular appearance, it could indicate general discomfort or pain.

Tone, speech patterns, and word choice can be indicators of mood. Think about the words the person is using in conversation to describe the subject matter. Do the words correspond with a positive or negative outlook, and what is this telling you? Is the care recipient more talkative, showing excitement or anxiety, or less talkative, possibly revealing they are angry or sad? Is the care recipient talking softly because he or she is depressed or tired, or talking loudly because he or she is mad or excited? Are the responses short, snappy, and abrupt, or is the care recipient taking time to carefully explain his or her point of view? Is the speech fast, slow, slurred, or incomprehensible?

If there is a persistent sad or depressed mood, a care provider should ask questions and start a dialogue with the care recipient in addition to making observations and interpreting nonverbal messages. The care provider should discuss issues with family or other professionals if there are significant changes in a care recipient's disposition or if there is a severe mood problem.

Home and Personal Care Routines

The care provider must first observe how a care recipient approaches and accomplishes routine tasks before the care provider can notice changes in personal care routines and how the home is maintained. If a care recipient has physical limitations, it is likely that adaptive methods for completing tasks have already been assessed and are in place. A care recipient may not complete a task as the care provider would, but be careful when judging the care recipient's approach and consider the circumstances from his or her point of view.

The home care provider should make mental or written notes of how the care recipient completes a given task. This becomes valuable information at a later time when it is necessary to evaluate how client service needs have changed. The following household practices and personal care routines should be observed initially and monitored during ongoing visits. Care providers should become familiar with care recipients' routines. This is not meant to be an invasion of privacy; rather, it is a method to learn and understand styles, abilities, and areas where additional assistance should be arranged.

Make observations in the following routines:

Household

Laundry
Cooking
Food storage
Linen storage
Light cleaning (vacuuming, dusting, dishes)
Trash removal
Mail and newspaper retrieval
Pet and plant care
Paperwork storage and organization
Doors and windows that should be opened or locked
Emergency response system

Personal

How the care recipient maneuvers through the living space, with or without
    equipment (i.e., wheelchair, cane)
How adaptive and medical equipment, such as canes, walkers, wheelchairs,
    and oxygen, are used
How the care recipient gets in and out of the bed, shower, chair, or car
How the care recipient physically dresses and undresses, as well as style
    preferences
Meal preparation: Does the care recipient use an oven or microwave? Does
    he or she eat frozen foods, leftovers, or order carryout food?
Use of kitchen appliances, including sharp knives

Personal affects, such as jewelry or hairstyle

Use of eyeglasses, dentures, hearing aids, and other sensory/functional enhancement equipment

Appointments and schedules: Does the care recipient have set weekly commitments?

Use of recreational and leisure time

It is useful to know how the care recipient spends purposeful and leisure time for a few reasons. Here, purposeful time implies the amount of time spent on Activities of Daily Living or Instrumental Activities of Daily Living, both serving to preserve an independent lifestyle. If a care recipient spends 3 hours getting dressed and preparing and eating breakfast, that may explain why he or she is tired for the rest of the afternoon and does not want to participate in recreational activities. The care provider can recommend related home care services, such as a home health aide to assist with personal care routines, to minimize this time the care recipient spends on daily routines. An excellent way to build rapport is to learn care recipients' hobbies and interests. A care provider may learn that in their spare time, a care recipient enjoys working picture puzzles. The care provider can use the picture's content to begin a conversation while working the puzzle with the care recipient during visits. To demonstrate attentiveness, a care provider may deliver puzzles to the care recipient. The puzzle becomes a tool for assessing functionality, and the leisure activity becomes a measuring stick. As with other routines, activities are a point of reference for measuring motivation, interest, and performance, and to observe behavior or mental changes. If, over time, it is noticed that the client becomes confused by the puzzle pieces or is no longer interested in working puzzles, the cognitive or emotional changes should be reported to family and other care providers.

Many people have distinctive habits and techniques for tending to themselves and household chores and organization. Sally eats only half her dinner in order to have leftovers rather than needing to prepare the next day's lunch. Joan insists on using butter instead of mayonnaise in her weekly bowl of egg salad, and Betty cannot sleep in her bed unless the sheet's fold line is down the middle of the mattress! Care providers must suspend any judgment of such unique practices; it is more important to meet care recipients' needs on their terms. They are paying for the service and it is this assistance that may keep them living independently longer. It is careful attention to client requests and demands that distinguish quality home care from care at home.

Eating and Sleeping Habits

A care provider may not have an opportunity to witness a care recipient's sleeping or eating habits, and may have to rely on verbal information that the care recipient offers. The care provider's objective is to determine if the care recipient is eating, and eating nutritionally, and if he or she is getting enough sleep; also, to note if there are changes in eating and sleeping patterns. Furthermore, being informed of meal and sleep times may affect the care provider's schedule; knowing the best time of day to visit so that your presence does not interfere with the care recipient's habits will result in more productive time spent together.

How can home care providers tell that the care recipient is eating or sleeping if they are not present during meals or regular sleep times? It would seem obvious if a person is not getting enough sleep: He or she may not feel up to any activity, will be habitually tired, and take frequent naps. The care provider should be aware if the care recipient is not sleeping enough or getting too much sleep, as either could be symptoms of a medical condition. It may be easier to monitor care recipients' eating habits than sleep patterns. If a job duty of the care provider is to grocery shop for or with the care recipient, the care provider can monitor the types of food purchased for nutritional value, and the amounts eaten between trips to the grocery store.

Changes in Pain or Discomfort

The care provider should help the care recipient to be more comfortable, but should know when to ask medical professionals (nurses, doctors, and therapists) to intervene. It is not the home care provider's role to treat pain, yet it is a responsibility to report to family and health professionals when the care recipient is experiencing changes in level of pain as well as the effectiveness of pain medications. Is the medicine managing symptoms? Is the care recipient taking extra doses to manage the pain? Notice when the care recipient is feeling more or less pain. Does it depend on how the care recipient is positioned? Are there certain times of the day, or even of the year, when more pain is experienced? (People with arthritis feel stiffer during wet and humid weather.) Is there a connection between episodes of pain and emotionally difficult conversations or decisions that may promote lifestyle changes? As with other observations, care providers should communicate the changes in pain levels to other professionals involved in care.

The above is a basic list of areas for practicing observation skills. They are also starting points for understanding the bigger picture of the caregiving situation so that the care provider can prepare for scheduled visits by knowing what type of assistance will be needed. The care provider will understand the working circumstances and have a general knowledge of what to expect during subsequent visits by examining and evaluating these five areas on the first visit with a care recipient. To gain further insight into the care recipient and caregiving situation, use the five senses: hearing, seeing, smelling, tasting, and touching. An often-overlooked sense is intuition, which companions and caregivers use regularly and label as, "I just knew." The following examples show how to use the senses for a deeper understanding of what is or is not being said.

Hearing

Do some subjects tend to frustrate the client, in which case they talk louder? The care provider should notice if and when the voice volume or tone change, either getting louder or softer. Is the voice raised, possibly indicating they do not like the food they see in front of them? Or maybe they do not want to eat? Is the client using a calm voice and appearing delighted to eat the meal? Do other subjects sadden the client and you notice that their voice lowers, becoming quieter? Does the client sound angry or pleased? Consider the choice of words the client is using to describe the subject matter. Do the words fit into the conversation or does it sound as if they are referring to another issue? People with Alzheimer's disease or other dementia tend to lose nouns from their vocabulary, often using incorrect words in descriptions. A couch may be called a car or a car may be called a building; otherwise, the content may be appropriate and fitting. Pay attention to the context and look around for visual clues of what the client is seeing. If he or she is sitting at the dining table and pointing to the plate but call it a bed, chances are they are really referring to the plate. Listen with carefulness.

Seeing

Upon contact with the care recipient, the care provider should take a visual inventory beginning with physical appearance. Does the care recipient look clean and well-groomed? Does his or her presence appear normal for them or do they look more disheveled? The care provider should monitor if the care recipient seems tired and apathetic or rested and involved throughout the visit. Be aware of the physical environment. Is there enough light in the room? Do throw rugs or electrical cords pose a risk of falling to the care recipient? Is the room cluttered or picked up? Are there spills that need to be cleaned up? In caregiving situations, what the care provider observes is valuable information because many times the client may not think or know to share subtle or even obvious issues. The care provider should be aware if the care recipient uses any adaptive or medical equipment and watch how he or she performs particular personal and household routines. These observations will become helpful in the future if the care provider begins to observe changes in physical or cognitive functioning.

Smelling

Is there an unusual odor when you walk into the environment? Does the client have an unclean smell? Is the client aware of the unusual odor? If a client lives in any type of independent living situation, check the refrigerator and trash cans. The client may not be physically able to take out the trash regularly and may need assistance. Many people store leftover food and keep perishables for too long, resulting in rotten or spoiled food. Care recipients may be unable to reach some areas of the refrigerator, cabinets, or even counters to throw away rotten foods. It is common for food to be left in the microwave, forgotten before or even after it was cooked. When unusual smells are noticed, take time to look and find the source.

Tasting

It should not be a regular practice to eat clients' food, but there may be times tasting foods for temperature and flavor (i.e., too salty or too sweet) is necessary.

There is no need to taste foods with an odor; the safest measure is to throw away the items. When working with care recipients who are confused or have slow reaction time, tasting or touching food to see if it is too hot or too cold can prevent harm. If a confused care recipient will not eat, sampling the food for flavor may help the care provider understand why the care recipient is not eating. A care provider regularly added sugar to the care recipient's water because that was the only way the care recipient, with Alzheimer's disease, would drink water. Care providers should use good judgment: Not every meal offering needs to be tasted, and certainly not when the care provider or recipient has a communicable illness or virus.

Touching

Be aware of care recipients' sensitivity and tolerance of affection; some people are guarded with their personal space and do not like to be touched. Yet, there may be reasons why touching a care recipient is necessary beyond assisting with transfers or mobility, such as when the sense of touch is useful for assessing a situation. A care recipient may need to be touched for temperature to determine if he or she is too hot or too cold, or if a wound or bruise is hard or soft. Other objects may need to be touched, such as an iron or stove to feel if it is warm, or touching the carpet or floor to feel if it is wet. It may be as simple as touching potted plants to determine if they need water. (This may be requested by the care recipient or can be an extra touch of comfort the care provider can offer.) If the care provider shops for a care recipient, touch similar fabrics and materials, which can help the care provider understand the care recipient's request for a needed item.

Intuition

We use the traditional five senses to gather information, and use that information to assess situations to then form assumptions. We draw on familiar experiences with similar circumstances to organize our perceptions and find related answers. Intuition is the ability to know without the use of logical methods that mysteriously works its way into situations. The power of intuition is recognized when it is said, "I just had a feeling," or "My hunch is . . ." We feel validated when the experience results in being correct. It is not to be an exercise of self-righteousness; the knowledge and experience should be used to guide future practices of problem solving and decision making. Intuition is used in problem-solving situations when there are unknowns, as well as in decision making when there is known factual information.

Using intuition and our five senses expands our perception beyond a one-dimensional approach and gives the ability to interpret experiences and situations by observing what is not always verbalized (see Tip 4.1). Changes in client actions and behaviors will become recognizable when nonverbal observations are determined during early visits. Significant to caregiving situations is not only the unique or particular way a person manages a task, but also how managing these tasks changes over time—possibly indicating the need for more or other assistance due to physical, mental, or cognitive changes.

Tip 4.1

What Is the Client Telling You?

1. When you walk into your client's apartment, you immediately notice toast on the floor, an overturned yogurt container on the table, an untouched glass of juice on the counter, and dish towels on the kitchen floor. The client is asleep on the couch nearby with her shirt buttoned haphazardly and a blanket covering her bare legs. A couple of pill bottles and the telephone are on the coffee table in front of the couch.

   Possibilities

   The client prepared a small meal but did not eat some or most of it
   The client did not get enough sleep or is feeling ill
   Spills or other messes occurred on the kitchen floor and the client had trouble cleaning up
   The client had difficulty getting dressed
   There was an incident of incontinence and the client did not put pants on afterwards
   The client took medications that could be affecting functioning
   The client tried calling someone or is waiting for a phone call

2. Every Tuesday morning, you assist a client with errand running and light home maintenance. She is always dressed and wearing lipstick and rouge. Regularly she is sitting in her wheelchair or electric lift chair reading the newspaper. The grocery list is in the usual place, on the kitchen table, with coupons, money, and a prescription.

   Possibilities

   She is self-determined, alert, and organized
   She is independent with decision making and able to name food preferences
   She has some limitations but knows what she is capable of managing
   Her physical appearance and presentation are important
   She continues to be interested in the outside world and current events
   She takes the time and effort to cut coupons out of the newspaper, and is therefore aware of product offerings and saving money
   In advance, she considers what amount of money she will need and the purpose for spending
   She is conscious of her medication supply

3. You arrive at the client's (in #2, above, who is usually well dressed), but she is still in her nightclothes, hair uncombed, and breakfast is still in the microwave. She cannot find her coupons and does not have a grocery

list. She is disorganized and uninterested, which is a noticeable change from previous visits.

Possibilities

Something has occurred that created these changes since your last visit

She was up during the night and did not get enough sleep

She is not feeling well

She has not eaten, which could be affecting her functioning

She could be over- or undermedicated

She is depressed

There are two important reasons for making good observations. The first is to understand care recipient habits, preferences, and styles to provide the type of individualized care that the client deserves. A goal of home health services is to deliver customized care and comfort into the care recipient's home to promote aging in place, where the care recipient remains in the familiar environment to preserve regular routines, with as little as possible disruption to lifestyle. The relationship will not develop and the care recipient may terminate service if a care provider forces his or her methodologies or significantly changes care recipient routines. The second reason is to establish a benchmark, or baseline, of behaviors and routines to recognize changes in attitude and approach. It doesn't matter if the care recipient sleeps in every morning until 10:00 a.m. What matters is when the care provider notices that the care recipient is now waking up every morning at 8:00 a.m. or sleeping until noon. Well-balanced meals are important to good health, but changing eating habits to raw vegetables and fruit will be difficult when the care recipient is accustomed to eating prepared or frozen foods. What should be noted is if the care recipient stops eating favored foods or changes the amount (more or less) of consumption. There are plenty of observations to make with varying degrees of significance and intensity; consider what is worthy of attention while realizing that situations can change—what is important now may not be over time and other circumstances may take priority. Being aware, alert, and observant will make information available that helps the companion provide quality care.

Summary

Patience, understanding, and flexibility are common characteristics of companions and caregivers. In addition, good communication skills are important for establishing rapport with a client, building relationships, understanding client wants and needs, and relaying accurate information to family members and other professionals. Well-developed communication skills build better working relationships, resulting in deeper human connections and quality client care. Knowledge and practice for improving conversation and listening, as well as problem-solving, decision-making, and conflict-resolutions skills, will develop versatile personal and professional abilities. Being better skilled in interpersonal communications enhances job productivity and performance as well as deepens interactions and relationships with others.

Perceived and real family roles can add tension in caregiving situations. A care provider may not be made aware of the history of family relationships. Advocating client needs is appropriate and care providers should avoid taking sides in family disputes. They must use good judgment so as to not get involved with challenging family dynamics.

A care provider receives verbal and nonverbal information that is interpreted to meet care recipient and family needs and expectations. The use of sensory perceptions—hearing, seeing, tasting, smelling, and touching—is necessary to recognize nonverbal messages. These subtle or obvious observations can be useful for evaluating how care recipients' strengths and weaknesses have changed over time. Changes in care recipient behaviors may be a sign of the need for more or other assistance, or a change in their physical and cognitive functioning.

Questions

What is meant by interpersonal skills?

How does a person communicate effectively?

Name three barriers to effective communications.

What is the importance of observing nonverbal communications?

What are reasons a care recipient may be reluctant to share information?

Why is it important for a care provider to understand personal perceptions?

What are sources of family tension and conflict?

What should be observed in caregiving situations? How should this be accomplished?

Summary Tips

Asking enough questions to comprehend a situation from another person's point of view leads to a deeper understanding of needs and concerns and aids in finding effective solutions.

Avoiding conflict is the best approach in caregiving situations.

Using your five senses provides a framework for observing what is not being verbalized and adding depth to what is being verbalized.

Helpful Web Sites

Articles for improving communication and interpersonal skills: American Management Association at http://www.amanet.com

Resources for improving career skills: http://www.mindtools.com

Resources and how-to guides for successful relations: http://www.inc.com

Suggested Reading

Bolton, Robert. (1986). *People skills: How to assert yourself, listen to others, and resolve conflicts*. New York: Simon and Schuster Adult Publishing Group. Communication-skills handbook outlining the 12 most common communication barriers.

DeVito, Joseph. (2007). *Interpersonal messages: Communication and relationship skills*. Upper Saddle River, NJ: Allyn and Bacon. How to build interpersonal communication skills.

Gladwell, Malcolm. (2007). *Blink: The power of thinking without thinking*. New York: Little, Brown and Company. Psychology and the process of decision making.

Klein, Gary A. (2002). *Intuition at work: Why developing your gut instincts will make you better at what you do*. New York: Doubleday Publishing. How the "gut feeling" and patterns of recognition influence decision making.

Common Conditions and Diseases of the Aging Body

5

In This Chapter, You Will Learn

1. A basic knowledge of age-related conditions and diseases: facts, symptoms, and treatments

2. Contact information for furthering education about specific diseases and conditions

3. Disease-specific roles and responsibilities of the care provider

Why This Matters

The natural mental, physical, and physiological processes of aging are different for every person during any stage of development. Not every person with Alzheimer's disease or suffering from a stroke will experience the exact same signs and symptoms; nor will each person receive or respond to the same treatment options. Care providers should be educated about the facts, signs, symptoms, and treatment options of diseases common to the aging population. However, over time, working with the older population will present similar circumstances and conditions even if outcomes vary. These experiences will be helpful to home care providers, who can offer suggestions based on previous practice and knowledge. Cognitive Psychologist Gary Klein (2003) states,

As we work in any area we accumulate experiences and build up a reservoir of recognized patterns. The more patterns we learn, the easier it is to match a new situation to one of the patterns in our reservoir. When a new situation occurs, we recognize the situation as familiar by matching to a pattern we have encountered in the past. (p. 11)

Care providers can use prior experience and intuition when managing health situations and organizing adaptive living conditions. The blending of education and experience gives the home care provider a larger knowledge base to explore more possibilities for better, individualized care.

The Aging Body

Consider this: For as long as you can remember, your favorite dinner was spaghetti. When you reach 74 years of age and eat a tomato-based sauce or other tomato-based dishes, your throat becomes irritated and you experience heartburn with a burning sensation in your stomach. The doctor finally diagnoses you with Gastroesophageal Reflux Disease (known as GERD) and recommends that you change your diet and take over-the-counter medicines to treat the symptoms. Foods rich in acids—tomatoes—and fats are restricted. You decide that eating foods that aggravate your symptoms is not worth the physical discomfort; to minimize or eliminate symptoms, you drastically alter your diet by eating bland, unspicy, low-fat foods. The new diet consists of cereals, grains, vegetables, and limited meat servings. You can no longer eat spaghetti, whole milk, oranges, hamburgers, and fast food; worst of all, chocolate is not tolerated with conditions from GERD! After decades of eating enjoyable and relatively healthy foods (milk, tomatoes, fruits), you now make conscious decisions about which foods you can and cannot eat and think about how every bite of food will interact with your bodily systems.

As the body ages, physical, physiological, and mental processes change. The body may not tolerate foods, medications, stimulation, or physical activity the way it once did, forcing a person to adapt to new routines and methods for coping. Lifelong habits may no longer be effective and there must be a search for new solutions, usually through trial and error. This process and adjustment can be stressful and even saddening, as the person experiencing such changes may feel a sense of loss and grief.

There are conditions and illnesses that develop with more frequency in older years. This chapter highlights 23 age-related conditions and diseases with an overview of facts, signs and symptoms, and common treatments. This information is not intended to be medical advice; it is meant to provide basic information that care providers may encounter when working with the elderly population. Contact information for national organizations to obtain condition- and disease-specific information is also provided. Suggested roles and responsibilities of the care provider are offered with tips for providing quality care and service.

Though particular recommendations are given for managing condition- and disease-specific situations, there are general actions a care provider should take:

Follow medical advice
Assist the care recipient in following medical advice

Become educated about care recipient's conditions

Educate the care recipient as needed with disease-specific knowledge and facts

Inform family, physician, or health care professionals of changes in care recipient's conditions

Encourage care recipients or family to attend support groups as appropriate

Be supportive, flexible, and compassionate

The care provider should not advise care recipients on medical decisions, though they should be educated in conditions, symptoms, and treatment options. The role of the care provider is to listen empathetically and be supportive of the care recipient. A genuine understanding of care recipients' situations creates compassion, and requires being educated to the medical and psychological circumstances and then sensitive to the significant decision-making processes that will follow. These general guidelines will promote excellence from the care provider, ultimately enhancing service delivery for quality care.

Alcoholism

Alcoholism is dependence on alcohol, which can affect a person's health, home, work, and social relationships. The National Institute on Alcohol Abuse and Alcoholism (NIAAA) defines alcoholism as a disease that includes the following symptoms:

Craving—a strong need to drink

Loss of control—the inability to stop drinking once a person has started

Physical dependence—withdrawal symptoms, such as nausea, sweating, and shakiness

Tolerance—the need to drink larger amounts of alcohol to feel the effects

Signs and Symptoms

Alcohol abuse may not be easily identifiable because many alcoholics hide their excessive use. This is a symptom of the disease. There are obvious signs that can indicate alcohol is a problem, which can be

Anxiety

Auto accidents or tickets related to alcohol

Blackouts/memory loss

Careless accidents

Depression

Difficulty with relationships

Hallucinations

Insomnia

Loss of self-esteem

Mood problems (typically with temper and anger management)

Poor work performance

Seizures
Trembling hands

Treatment

At this time, there is no cure for alcoholism though it can be treated. People with alcoholism are strongly encouraged not to drink to prevent a relapse, which can create additional problems. Alcoholism is treated with programs that use counseling and medications to help the person stop drinking. Other medications help minimize withdrawal symptoms such as shakiness, nausea, and sweating. An alcoholic or someone with a drinking problem should be encouraged to seek help from a physician, counselor, Alcoholics Anonymous, or other type of support group.

The Care Provider's Role and Responsibilities

If the care recipient is not already seeking help, encourage him or her to do so by attending AA meetings, seeking religious or spiritual counseling, or finding other types of support groups. Collect dates, times, and locations for meetings and provide the care recipient or family members with pertinent information. The care recipient should be educated about the disease and know how to seek help. The care provider should consult with a social worker, counselor, or other mental health professional for the best approach when working with an alcoholic client. These professionals should be involved especially if the care recipient or others are in danger or if safety is of concern. It is not the care provider's role or responsibility to perform any type of intervention; trained professionals should manage such situations.

More Information

Alcoholics Anonymous support groups are in most cities; check the yellow pages or online (http://www.aa.org) for local information. For disease-related information, contact NIAAA at:

National Institute on Alcohol Abuse and Alcoholism
5635 Fishers Lane, MSC 9304
Bethesda, MD 20892-9304
301-443-3860
http://www.niaaa.nih.gov

Alzheimer's Disease

Alzheimer's is the most common cause of dementia. Alzheimer's is a degenerative brain disease that eventually erases a person's memory and ability to learn, think, communicate, make decisions, and perform daily activities. As the disease progresses, changes in personality, mood, and behavior appear. Anxiety and agitation are common symptoms of this disease, while other people may become pleasantly confused. There is no way to predict how an affected person will progress with the disease.

Memory problems can be a normal part of aging. The Alzheimer's Association (2007b) makes these distinctions between normal age-related memory problems and the possibility of Alzheimer's disease:

Alzheimer's symptoms

Forgets entire experiences
Rarely remembers later
Gradually unable to follow oral/written directions
Gradually unable to use notes as reminders

Normal age-related memory changes

Forgets part of an experience
Often remembers later
Usually able to follow written or spoken directions
Usually able to care for the self

Barry Reisberg, MD, Clinical Director of the New York University School of Medicine Silberstein's Aging and Dementia Research Center, developed the Global Deterioration Scale (GDS) from which the Seven Stages of Alzheimer's is derived (see Tip 5.1). The model is based on expert research of common patterns found in effected individuals (Alzheimer's Association, 2007a).

Tip 5.1

The Seven Stages of Alzheimer's

Stage 1: No impairment

Signs of the disease are not evident to the person or any health care professional.

Stage 2: Very mild decline

The person experiences some memory loss that can appear as difficulty remembering names and misplacing keys, glasses, and other frequently used objects. The signs are not present in a medical examination and family and friends do not detect a problem.

Stage 3: Mild decline

It is this stage that family and friends could notice memory problems, which may be identified in medical examinations and tests. The affected person may be unable to recall words and names, have difficulties with recent short-term memory and concentration, noticeable performance changes in the workplace or in daily routines, and have trouble planning or organizing.

Stage 4: Moderate decline (mild or early stage)

In this stage, a medical evaluation will detect obvious deficiencies. The person with Alzheimer's has less memory of personal information and less short term memory of recent events. The ability to perform mental tasks, such as paying bills and managing finances, is challenging. The person may need assistance with IADLs. Even social situations can be challenging and the person may become withdrawn.

Stage 5: Moderately severe decline (moderate or mid-stage)

Decline in cognitive functioning and memory recall may interfere with daily activities and routines in this stage and assistance will be necessary. The person will be confused to day, time and season, and may not be able to dress appropriately to the weather or occasion. The ability to remember important information, such as their address, phone number, and other personal details is impaired. Usually, a person in this stage will know their own name as well as their spouse and children. Also, a person usually does not require assistance with eating or toileting.

Stage 6: Severe decline (moderately severe or mid-stage)

Cognitive impairment and memory problems get worse, personality changes will become apparent, and assistance with ADLs (dressing and toileting) is needed. Short-term memory skills are severely impaired and the person has difficulty recalling personal history information. Faces may be familiar, but the person can forget the names of a spouse, children, or other caregivers. The person may confuse day and night sleep schedules in this stage and incontinence becomes an issue. Behavior and personality issues arise, and the person may experience delusions and hallucinations. Repetitive behaviors, such as hand-wringing and pacing may appear.

Stage 7: Very severe decline (severe or late stage)

In this final stage of the disease, the person gradually loses control of the body. They require assistance with all ADLs (eating, dressing, toileting, and eventually walking). The ability to speak and to comprehend is gradually lost. The person appears to not be aware of the environment and may not respond to stimuli.

Note: Copyright 1983 by Barry Reisberg, MD. Reproduced with permission.

Signs and Symptoms

The Alzheimer's Association has created a list of 10 general warning signs to the possibility of Alzheimer's disease:

Memory loss
Difficulty performing familiar tasks

Problems with language
Disorientation to time and place
Poor or decreased judgment
Problems with abstract thinking
Misplacing things
Changes in mood or behavior
Changes in personality
Loss of initiative

Treatment

At this time, there is no cure for Alzheimer's disease. There are medications available that appear to slow down the disease process. Other medications are used to treat symptoms of the disease. For example, a person with Alzheimer's disease who experiences depression or anxiety may be prescribed antidepressants or antianxiety medicines, which do not actually treat the disease.

At least initially, nonmedication interventions are strongly encouraged. This requires patience and effort from family, friends, and other caregivers. It is important to identify the behavior, understand the cause, and adapt the environment or situation to meet personal and safety needs to manage behaviors. A nondrug approach is about managing issues and concerns, not trying to change or correct the affected person's behaviors. Being argumentative and confrontational is not productive and escalates the situation. The best approach is to keep matters easy to understand and redirect the person's attention away from distressing and complicated issues.

There are two recommended forms of therapeutic communications that benefit people with Alzheimer's (and other dementias): Reality Orientation and Validation Therapy. These techniques encourage participation at the level of the care recipients' ability. *Reality Orientation* uses verbal and visual reminders and repetition to orient a person to current surroundings: day, time, and season, as well as familiar people, places, and events. *Validation Therapy* respects the reality of the affected person by suspending judgment; instead of making corrections, words and thoughts should be accepted regardless of accuracy or appropriateness. Asking questions (who, what, when, where, and how) helps the person feel heard, giving confidence and promoting a sense of safety. Appropriate use of Reality Orientation and Validation Therapy is dependent on what stage the care recipient is in of the disease process. Based on experience, a general rule of thumb is: If it is frustrating or upsetting to reorient a person to the current reality, simply validate their perspective to avoid any confrontation or distressing situation.

The Care Provider's Role and Responsibilities

Until a care provider gains experience, Alzheimer's education—expected behaviors, changes, and progression—is invaluable. The care provider must be patient, flexible, and understanding with the Alzheimer's person, who is doing the best that he or she can do. Duties may include assistance, supervision, and suggestions for simplifying daily routines. Most importantly, the care provider should focus on making the care recipient comfortable by eliminating stressors and sources of frustration. The care provider's role is to provide companionship and become a source of comfort to the person with the disease.

The care provider also acts as a support to the family. Encouraging family members to become educated about the disease is very important so that they may better understand physical, mental, and cognitive changes. Also, suggest that family attend local support group meetings and provide family members with meeting dates, times, and locations.

More Information

Alzheimer's Association (National Office)
225 N. Michigan Ave., Floor 17
Chicago, IL 60601
800-272-3900
http://www.alz.org

Arthritis

Arthritis is commonly thought of as an older person's condition, though it occurs in people of all ages. It can cause pain, stiffness, and swelling in the joints, making daily activities difficult to accomplish. Many people live with arthritis for years; it is usually a chronic (ongoing) condition. There are different types of arthritis, but rheumatoid and osteoarthritis are most common to the elderly population. Rheumatoid arthritis is inflammation of the joints, which can lead to limited mobility and range of motion. Osteoarthritis is the breakdown of cartilage around the bones, leading to pain and swelling in the knees, hips, lower back, neck, hands, and feet. The Arthritis Foundation states that osteoarthritis rarely affects other joints except as the result of an injury (Arthritis Foundation, 2006, p. 2).

Signs and Symptoms

Arthritis symptoms vary from person to person but are usually identified by pain and the inability to complete daily activities, swelling, stiffness, and difficulty moving a joint. A person with rheumatoid arthritis can have warm, swollen, and painful joints, evidenced by pinkness on the skin's surface. Affected joints will be stiff and painful when they are not used. People with osteoarthritis find it difficult to move in the morning and after too much use of a joint.

Treatment

Arthritis is managed, not cured. Many people take medications to reduce the swelling and pain. Weight control can help relieve pressure that causes pain. Exercise and physical and occupational therapies are often part of the management plan to improve range of motion and muscle strength. Another treatment is heat and cold therapy as directed by a physician or physical or occupational therapist. Braces, splints, canes, and walkers are also used to assist with mobility and flexibility.

The Care Provider's Role and Responsibilities

Usually, roles and responsibilities are assisting the care recipient with physical tasks that they may no longer be able to perform, or that are too time consuming for the care recipient. Chores around the home or errand running are typical duties. This assistance with nonpersonal care routines may give the care recipient the additional time that it takes to perform other measures of self-care, making it feasible for the care recipient to remain living independently. Care recipients are typically well aware of how arthritis is affecting their abilities and restricting movements, though getting information about the disease could be helpful. In the least, providing the care recipients with information may just show that the care provider is interested in care recipient issues and concerns.

More Information

The Arthritis Foundation
P.O. Box 7669
Atlanta, GA 30357-0669
800-568-4045
http://www.arthritis.org

Bedsores

A bedsore (also known as pressure ulcer, pressure wound, or decubitus ulcer) is an open-skin area or wound on any part of the body. Bedsores are caused by continuous pressure to a particular part of the body often resulting from staying in one position for a prolonged period of time, such as in a bed or wheelchair, which restricts blood flow to that area. Bedsores regularly occur on the heels, legs, hips, arms or elbows, back, and buttocks. Exposure to moisture (such as lying in urine for too long) contributes to skin breakdown and increases the risk of bedsores.

Signs and Symptoms

There are four stages of bedsores determined by the severity and deepness of the open wound. An early sign of a pressure ulcer is redness, burning, swelling, and tenderness. The affected area may feel warm to the touch and the skin is not broken. It is in stage three that the skin opens and the wound settles deeper into the layers of skin. It is this stage when extreme care and attention is needed because the wound is susceptible to infection. If the wound becomes infected, it could enter stage four, meaning that the sore extends beyond the skin into muscle and tissue. If bedsores are not treated timely (earlier rather than later) they can cause sepsis and become life threatening.

Treatments

To prevent bedsores, good skin care is important. The affected area should be cleaned frequently to prevent infection and skin should be well moisturized. A healthy diet with protein-rich foods is good for the skin and aids in healing open wound areas. A person should be out of bed as much as possible and as tolerated. If this is not possible, a regular schedule of turning and repositioning is important for keeping the skin clean and to minimize pressure on the same areas. Pillows, sheepskin, and other padding can be used to position the person off of the affected area. Special ointments and dressings may be used in the healing process and antibiotics will be needed if the wound becomes infected. In a wound's later stages, surgical procedures are necessary to clean out the infection, known as de-breeding. The best approach for managing bedsores is prevention.

The Care Provider's Role and Responsibilities

The care provider can be very helpful in monitoring the healing or worsening of pressure ulcers. There will be obvious physical signs and any areas of concern should be reported to the nurse, physician, or other professional providing care. A care provider can also help by seeing that the care recipient is eating a healthy diet, encouraging protein-rich foods. A nurse or physical therapist may instruct the care provider on proper positioning techniques for keeping the care recipient physically comfortable. It is not recommended that a care provider treat any open wounds. Doctors, nurses, and wound-care specialists should manage medications and apply ointments or bandage dressings.

More Information

Medline Plus (a service of the U.S. National Library of Medicine and the National Institutes of Health) at http://www.nlm.nih.gov/medlineplus/pres suresores.html

Cancer

Cancer is not contagious. A normal physiological process of the body is to form new cells that replace old cells that die. Sometimes, new cells grow when they are not needed and old cells do not die when they should, which results in extra cells. These cells can form a mass, known as a tumor, which can be benign (not cancerous) or malignant (cancerous). Cells from the malignant tumors overrun surrounding tissue, or can spread into other parts of the body through the lymph or blood system. When the malignant cells grow and multiply throughout the body, it is called metastasis.

Signs and Symptoms

Most cancers are named because of where they start in the body. (For example, lung cancer starts in the lungs, as throat, breast, and ovarian cancers begin in these respective areas of the body.) Signs and symptoms of specific cancers depend on the type of cancer and how far advanced the disease is. Some people live a long time without knowing they have cancer.

The National Cancer Institute (2007) does identify possible signs of cancer:

A lump in the breast or other part of the body
An obvious change in the appearance of an existing mole or wart
A sore that does not heal
Hoarseness or a nagging cough
Changes in bowel or bladder habits
Difficulty swallowing
Persistent indigestion
Unexplained changes in weight (gain or loss)
Unusual bleeding or discharge

These are not automatic signs of cancer. It is imperative to consult a physician for an examination and proper diagnosis. There are numerous types of cancers with varying causes, signs, symptoms, and treatments. Medical advice from oncology (cancer) specialists is critical for cancer-specific information.

Treatment

In general, treatments can be medications, hormone therapy, radiation, or chemotherapy. A physician may use any combination of these treatments, depending on several factors. Physicians consider where the cancer is in the body and how advanced the condition is to determine the best treatment plan. Medical professionals will also consider the person's general health, age, and family history of the disease.

Treatment is most successful with early detection. To help detect pre-cancer conditions, tests are available: mammography, pap, and sigmoidoscopy, to name a few. Alternative therapies, known as Complementary and Alternative Medicine (CAM), are becoming more common to treat cancer. Medical doctors and other health professionals use what is considered standard care, and alternative medicines or therapies, such as acupuncture, meditation, and herbal medicines, are treatments that are considered nonstandard care approaches in the medical field. Alternative therapies may be used to treat the disease or manage disease symptoms. A physician should be informed of any and all treatment methods. Many people are able to manage the disease and cope with cancer as a way of life with medications and lifestyle adjustments.

The Care Provider's Role and Responsibilities

The roles and responsibilities of the care provider will vary depending on the type and stage of the care recipient's cancer. In general, the care provider should be prepared to offer emotional support: The care recipient may just need a non-family member with whom to share feelings of anger, fear, and sadness. Responsibilities of the care provider may be to run errands, perform other home chores, monitor health status for changes, or provide the care recipient with one-on-one attention.

More Information

American Cancer Society
1599 Clifton Road Northeast
Atlanta, GA 30329
800-228-2345
http://www.cancer.org

Congestive Heart Failure (CHF)

This is a very common condition in the older population, and many live with it for years. With this condition, the heart is not working efficiently and the body is not receiving blood and oxygen as it should. The body will retain fluids that can build up in the lungs or cause swelling in the feet and ankles (called edema) when the heart does not pump enough blood.

Signs and Symptoms

Symptoms develop over weeks, months, and years, and will get worse if not treated. Symptoms can include confusion, shortness of breath, swelling of the ankles or legs, tiredness, and weight gain or bloating from fluid build-up.

Treatment

A physician will need to diagnose the problems and prescribe medications accordingly. A person with congestive heart failure will need to be under the care of a physician and may need to take heart medications and water pills to reduce fluid build-up. Heart surgery is required in some cases. A healthy diet that limits salt intake is usually recommended (American Heart Association, 2004a).

The Care Provider's Role and Responsibilities

Because people can live for years with CHF, the care provider's responsibilities will depend on the severity of conditions. The care provider may help the care recipient organize needed medical equipment and delivery routines, such as oxygen tanks. Physical tasks can become difficult for a person with CHF. It is likely that a care provider will need to assist with tasks that are tiring for the care recipient

More Information

American Heart Association (National Center)
7272 Greenville Avenue
Dallas, TX 75231
800-242-8721
http://www.americanheart.org

Constipation

Constipation is a common problem in adults over 65 years. It is a symptom, not a disease. As foods pass through the large intestine, the colon absorbs water from the foods. Constipation occurs when the colon muscles slow and the stool does not move quickly enough through the intestine. The National Institute of Health defines constipation as having three or fewer bowel movements a week.

Common causes of constipation are:

Not enough fiber in the diet
Lack of exercise or physical activity
Medications
Too much milk
Irritable Bowel Syndrome
Changes in life routines (pregnancy, travel, aging)
Laxative abuse
Ignoring the need to have a bowel movement
Dehydration
Specific diseases or conditions (stroke is the most common)
Other problems with intestinal functioning

Medications can also cause constipation, especially antidepressants, antacids with aluminum and calcium, anticonvulsants, anti-Parkinson's medicines, blood pressure medications, diuretics, iron supplements, and pain medications.

Some diseases and conditions that slow the movement of stools and cause constipation are:

Cancer
Diabetes
Hypothyroidism
Lupus
Multiple sclerosis
Parkinson's disease
Scleroderma
Spinal cord injuries
Stroke

Signs and Symptoms

Stools that are usually small, dry, and hard, can be difficult or painful to pass. Constipation is defined as having any of the following two symptoms for at least 12 weeks in the previous 12 months:

Straining during bowel movements
Lumpy or hard stool
Blood in stool
Bloating

Sensation of not completely eliminating
Sensation of blockage
Fewer than three bowel movements a week

Treatment

Preventing constipation is the best approach and can start with a healthy diet. Eating high-fiber foods, including fruits, vegetables, and whole grains, is a necessary precaution. Water and exercise are important to keep foods moving through the intestine. It is critical to have a bowel movement when the sensation occurs; voluntary nondefecating creates more blockage problems. Many people initially treat constipation with over-the-counter medications, typically with laxatives. Severe cases of constipation are treated with a colon test, barium enema x-ray, sigmoidoscopy, and colonoscopy. Treating constipation depends on the cause, severity, and duration of the condition. In most situations, a change in dietary and lifestyle habits will prevent and relieve symptoms.

The Care Provider's Role and Responsibilities

A care provider can educate a care recipient on foods that are known to help relieve symptoms and improve bowel functioning. If the care provider is responsible for picking up over-the-counter medicines, talk with the care recipient about the condition and discuss with the pharmacist to learn the best treatment for the given symptoms. Many people do not openly talk about this personal problem. A care provider may never know that a care recipient is constipated or having trouble with elimination.

More Information

American Gastroenterological Association (National Office)
4930 Del Ray Avenue
Bethesda, MD 20814
301-654-2055
http://www.gastro.org

Continence

Continence is the ability to control bladder and bowel functioning. As we age, bladder and kidney capacities decrease. The kidneys are unable to filter wastes as quickly and the bladder is unable to hold as much, which means more frequent urination. In health care, continence is commonly addressed by its opposite, incontinence, which is the inability to control urinary functioning or bowel functioning or both. The kidneys produce urine that the bladder holds until there is the opportunity to urinate; when there is a breakdown in any part of this system, incontinence can occur. Bowel and bladder problems can be the symptom of another disease or the result of weakened or overactive muscles. Incontinence can occur from urinary tract infections, vaginal infections, constipation, and certain medications (i.e., diuretics). Stress incontinence is a condition in which the bladder and pelvic muscles are weak and accidents occur due to coughing, sneezing, laughing, or any movement that puts stress on the bladder. An overactive bladder, also known as urge incontinence, is a condition of active muscles in which a person feels a strong urge to urinate. Alzheimer's, dementia, stroke, and Multiple Sclerosis can cause this type of incontinence. Mixed incontinence occurs when symptoms of both stress and urge incontinence are present, though one type may be more noticeable.

Incontinence occurs at any age as the result of some surgeries and pregnancies, but is very common with the aged population. Getting oneself to the bathroom in a timely manner is a regular problem for older adults with mobility issues. This is called functional incontinence. For example, arthritis may prohibit a person from moving quickly enough to get to the bathroom or remove clothing before urination starts. Also, someone with early dementia may forget to go to the bathroom until it becomes urgent.

Signs and Symptoms

Symptoms of bladder problems range from mild leaking to uncontrollable wetting or defecating.

Treatment

Many situations of incontinence are treatable and controllable. A physician may take blood and urine tests to measure how well the bladder is functioning. Treatment depends on the type and cause of the incontinence. More often than not, lifestyle habits are considered when choosing the best treatment option. There are several types of catheters used for different reasons to manage incontinence. The most frequently used is the Foley catheter, a plastic tube inserted into the bladder to drain the urine into a heavy plastic bag.

The National Association for Continence identifies three categories of treatment. Behavioral techniques include scheduled toileting routines, such as reminding the person to use the toilet every 2 hours. Bladder training is also scheduled toileting, but involves increasing the length of time between each trip to train the bladder to delay voiding. This has been effective in treating urge and mixed incontinence. Exercising pelvic muscles (known as Kegel exercises) is often recommended for stress and urge incontinence. The second category, pharmacologic therapy, treats incontinence with medications. Consult with a physician or pharmacist before taking over-the-counter medications. The last treatment option is surgery. There are different procedures depending on the type of the incontinence.

The Care Provider's Role and Responsibilities

Signs of continence issues may not be evident for a period of time if the care recipient knows how to manage the situation. Possible signs can be an increase in the amount of laundry, particularly undergarments and bed linens. The bathroom or bedroom may be visibly unclean and very likely there will be an odor. The care provider should approach the conversation about continence supplies and solutions with compassion and care. Suggestions may include panty liners or thicker pads that adhere to undergarments (similar to women's sanitary pads) for mild leaking. Disposable, pull-up undergarments (commonly referred to by the brand name, Depends) are suitable for men and women if elimination is moderate, more than minor leaking. Another suggestion to offer is disposable or nondisposable bed pads (sometimes referred to as "chuck pads"), which protect the bed from wetness and are available at home medical supply stores and pharmacies. The discussion of catheters is best addressed by a nurse or a physician.

More Information

National Association for Continence
P.O. Box 1019
Charleston, SC 29402-1019
843-377-0900
http://www.nafc.org

Dementia

A confused and forgetful older person many times is quickly and inaccurately diagnosed as having Alzheimer's disease. The fact is there are several dementias, each with unique characteristics. Dementia is a loss of mental functioning, such as language, memory, visual or spatial abilities, or judgments and decision making, that affects daily life. Dementia could be a symptom of another condition and not a disease. Dementia is a symptom of diseases such as Alzheimer's, Pick's, and Parkinson's, and can be a consequence of physical conditions, such as head injuries, nutritional deficiencies, urinary infections, or medication reactions. Especially in the older population, depression will look like dementia: A depressed older adult can be forgetful and confused. A preoccupation with rational or irrational thoughts and ideas can also appear as absentminded and forgetful. A person experiencing dementia-like symptoms should be examined and tested to determine if the symptoms are reversible.

Note: There are too many dementias to detail here. It is not necessary to know the signs and symptoms of specific dementias until care recipients have the diagnosis, and then it is helpful to learn about the specific dementia for appropriate treatment plans.

Signs and Symptoms

There are some general signs of dementia that come at varying levels of severity. Memory loss is the most obvious sign, though not every problem with forgetfulness means dementia. Forgetfulness, along with disorientation, language problems, and misplacing things, could be indicative of a larger problem. People with dementia may no longer have good judgment to process decisions related to daily activities and routines. Aware that their mental status is changing, a person could become more irritable and angry or depressed and apathetic. Some people with dementia experience positive or negative personality and mood changes.

Treatment

Any indication of dementia should be evaluated by a doctor to determine the cause. After an accurate diagnosis, the physician will be better able to prescribe appropriate medications and behavior treatment options.

The Care Provider's Role and Responsibilities

As with Alzheimer's disease, the care provider must be patient, flexible, and understanding. Duties will vary depending on the stage of the dementia and the care recipient's living situation, but may include assistance, supervision, and suggestions for simplifying daily routines. The care provider should focus on making the care recipient comfortable by eliminating stressors and sources of frustration. The care provider's role is to provide companionship and become a source of comfort to the person with dementia.

The care provider may also act as a support to the family and educate members about common behaviors associated with dementia. This will help all involved to better understand physical, mental, and cognitive changes in their loved one. Also, suggest that family attend local support group meetings and provide family members with meeting dates, times, and locations.

More Information

The Alzheimer's Association will provide supplementary information about dementias other than Alzheimer's disease, including Multi-Infarct Dementia, Lewy body dementia, Creutzfeldt-Jakob, and Huntington's, Pick's, and Parkinson's diseases. The National Library of Medicine and the National Institute of Health offer general information about dementia at http://www.medlineplus.com.

Alzheimer's Association (National Office)
225 N. Michigan Ave., Floor 17
Chicago, IL 60601
800-272-3900
http://www.alz.org

Depression

Depression is a very common condition in the aging population, though it is not considered a normal part of aging. It is normal for any person to feel sad or depressed after a major life transition, financial problems, or the death of a loved one, friend, or family member. Chronic illnesses common to aging, such as diabetes, heart conditions, stroke, Parkinson's, and Alzheimer's can also cause depression. Additionally, some medications can actually cause depression. People become depressed for very individualized reasons and for some, no reason at all. A depressed mood that interferes with daily routines or extends beyond a few weeks can be a sign of a more serious problem with depression.

Signs and Symptoms

A depressed elderly person often appears confused and forgetful. Unfortunately, too many older adults are inaccurately diagnosed with dementia when depression is the real problem. Many are quick to label symptoms of memory loss and confusion as a type of dementia and do not consider depression as a source of the problem. If a person is correctly treated for depression, dementia-like symptoms may disappear.

Common symptoms of a problem with depression can include:

Persistent sad or anxious mood
Reduced or increased appetite and significant changes in weight (gain or loss)
Changes in sleep habits (increase or decrease)
Loss of interest in activities that once brought pleasure
A general loss of interest in things; loss of energy
Restlessness or irritability
Difficulty concentrating, remembering, or making decisions
Feeling hopeless or worthless
Expressions of hopelessness and worthlessness
Thoughts and expressions of suicide or death

If a person experiences three or more of these symptoms for longer than 2 weeks, consult with a physician or mental health professional.

Treatment

Depression is treatable. The most common treatment is with antidepressant medications. Psychotherapy, in combination with medications, is also used. Trained therapists and mental health professionals provide psychotherapy to offer effective ways for managing and coping with difficult life events. A physician, mental health professional, and other health care providers should coordinate the best treatment plan for the individual.

The Care Provider's Role and Responsibilities

Depression is a disease, but many people in older generations perceive it as a flaw in character and emotional strength. If a care recipient who is depressed is not already medicated, he or she should be encouraged to talk to the physician about treatment options. In successful care provider–care recipient relationships, care providers can be a great form of therapy for care recipients with depression. Many families hire companions "so Mom or Dad has someone to talk to." This does not mean that a companion should attempt psychotherapy on a care recipient. The companion should provide support and compassion, using active listening skills to understand concerns and needs. Companions and care providers should create pleasant and engaging opportunities for care recipients to divert focus from stressors and sources of frustration. A care provider should never assume more responsibility than he or she is capable of providing when helping care recipients with depression; they must use good judgment and know personal and professional limits and boundaries. Care providers must accept that they cannot cure the problem. Medical or mental health professionals may need to be involved, especially if the care recipient is experiencing severe symptoms (see "Mental Health" in this chapter).

More Information

American Psychological Association
750 First Street, NE
Washington, DC 20002-4242
800-374-2721; 202-336-5500
http://www.apa.org/topics/aging

Diabetes

Diabetes is characterized by higher amounts of sugar (glucose) in the blood or urine as a result of the body's inability to produce or properly use insulin. Insulin is a hormone produced in the pancreas that converts glucose in the cells to energy and lowers the level of sugar in the blood. In Type 1 diabetes, the pancreas does not produce enough insulin or the body does not respond to the insulin. As a result, the blood-sugar level will become elevated. Type 2 diabetes is more common and occurs when the body is unable to properly use insulin or there may be an insulin deficiency.

An additional problem that arises with diabetes is *hyperglycemia,* a condition caused when the body has high blood sugar and not enough insulin is produced. *Hypoglycemia* occurs when the blood-sugar level is low. Both complications produce health risks. Finding the balance between high and low glucose levels can be challenging and may require constant monitoring.

Signs and Symptoms

Type 1 and Type 2 diabetes share common symptoms that include:

Being very thirsty
Urinating often
Feeling very hungry or tired
Losing weight without trying

Having sores that heal slowly
Having dry, itchy skin
Losing the feeling in your feet or having tingling in your feet
Having blurry eyesight

Treatment

Keeping blood sugar and glucose levels close to the normal range is essential to reduce the risk of significant problems and long-term complications. Many diabetics test their blood sugar levels at least once a day to then carefully regulate insulin, exercise, and diet. Most diabetics inject themselves with insulin amounts determined by a physician. Diabetes is a chronic disease; like arthritis, it is managed but not cured, often requiring significant changes in lifestyle, behaviors, and habits. When sugar levels are controlled, most diabetics are able to live a productive life. Because diabetes can be a complex condition and potentially life threatening, it is extremely important to visit the physician regularly and as needed for any individualized treatment plans.

The Care Provider's Role and Responsibilities

The care provider's role assisting diabetic care recipients can range from monitoring that meals are eaten regularly, ensuring that insulin and other medications are taken and blood sugar is checked routinely, to planning and preparing appropriate meals, grocery shopping, and other necessary errands. Also, supplies (lancets, glucose monitoring devices) may need to be ordered on a regular schedule. Discuss with the care recipient, family, or other involved health care professional who is responsible for ensuring these supplies are available to the care recipient. Diabetics with more severe conditions may have other needs and demands; be sure to clearly understand care recipient and family expectations.

More Information

American Diabetes Association
1701 North Beauregard Street
Alexandria, VA 22311
800-342-2383
http://www.diabetes.org

Gastroesophageal Reflux Disease (GERD)

Though GERD occurs in people of all ages, it is important to include because of the dietary guidelines that change for a person with the condition. GERD is a chronic condition in which digestive juices regurgitate from the stomach into the esophagus, the tube that transports food and liquids from the mouth to the stomach. With GERD, the valve between the esophagus and stomach may open spontaneously or does not close properly; when it malfunctions, foods and fluids are tasted in the mouth and may cause a burning sensation in the throat or chest, known as heartburn. Reflux disease is diagnosed as GERD if the problem occurs more than twice a week. The causes of GERD are unknown, though research indicates that having a hiatal hernia, which allows acid reflux to occur more easily, may contribute to GERD. According to research, GERD may contribute to asthma, a chronic cough, or pulmonary fibrosis.

Signs and Symptoms

In adults, the most common symptom is frequent heartburn—a burning sensation or pain in the lower part of the midchest, behind the breastbone, and in the midabdomen. Heartburn does not always indicate GERD and some people may have GERD without heartburn.

Treatment

The National Institute of Diabetes and Digestive and Kidney Diseases offers treatment suggestions of lifestyle changes, medications, and when necessary, surgery. Recommended lifestyle changes are to

Stop smoking
Avoid foods and drinks that worsen symptoms
Lose weight, if needed
Eat small, frequent meals
Wear loose-fitting clothes
Avoid lying down for 3 hours after eating
Raise the head of the bed 6–8 inches; using extra pillows will not help

A pharmacist or physician can recommend over-the-counter antacids that relieve heartburn symptoms; common brands are Alka-Seltzer, Rolaids, Mylanta, and Maalox. Additional medications can be used to treat the linings of the throat or stomach, and there are other medications used to improve muscle functioning in the digestive tract. A physician should monitor any medication routines used to manage symptoms of GERD for drug interactions and effectiveness. If symptoms do not improve, a physician may recommend further testing to determine the need for surgery.

The Care Provider's Role and Responsibilities

The care provider can provide information and education on how to manage the symptoms of GERD, possibly suggesting diet alternatives and food choices that will improve symptoms. If the care provider does the grocery shopping, he or she should consider which foods may aggravate symptoms. Additionally, it may be the care provider who talks to the pharmacist or physician about the symptoms and he or she will need to relay accurate information between the health care professionals and the care recipient.

More Information

National Digestive Disease Information Clearing House
(presented by The National Institute of Diabetes and Digestive and Kidney
    Diseases)
2 Information Way
Bethesda, MD 20892-3570
800-891-5389
http://www.digestive.niddk.nih.gov

Hearing Loss

A permanent hearing loss happens when there is damage to the inner ear or
auditory nerve. A temporary loss of hearing can occur when sound waves cannot reach the inner ear because of wax buildup, fluid, or a punctured eardrum.
This temporary loss is treatable, but if left untreated can cause further problems or a permanent loss of hearing. Some people experience loss of only certain sounds and pitches while others may lose all hearing.

Hearing loss can be hereditary, or the result of a trauma, infection, or reactions to certain medications. A loss of hearing can occur at any age, especially if
a person is subject to environmental factors that impact hearing, such as regular exposure to loud noises. Many older adults lose at least part of their hearing
abilities. Presbycusis is a common form of hearing loss in people over 50 years
because of changes in the inner ear, auditory nerve, middle ear, or outer ear.

Signs and Symptoms

Tinnitus is another common symptom of hearing loss in older adults, which is
described as ringing, hissing, or roaring sounds in the ears. Exposure to loud
noise or certain medicines can cause tinnitus. Other signs of hearing loss may
be any combination of three or more of the following:

Trouble hearing over the telephone
Trouble hearing when there is background noise or more than one conver-
    sation occurring at a time
Straining to hear or understand a conversation
Misunderstanding what others are saying and therefore responding inap-
    propriately
Asking others to repeat themselves
Others complain that television or radio volumes are too loud

Treatment

There are ways to manage the effects of hearing loss when it is not reversible.
Hearing aids come in a variety of sizes, shapes, and styles. An audiologist can
evaluate and determine if hearing aids are the best approach. An otolaryngologist (a surgeon who specializes in ear, nose, and throat conditions) should be

consulted for the possibility of an ear implant. Implants do not restore hearing; rather, they help the person understand some speech. A speech language pathologist and audiologist will provide assistance with this learning process. Technological advances are constantly developing devices for telephones, televisions, and other household appliances to reduce background noise or create visual—in addition to auditory—signals.

The Care Provider's Role and Responsibilities

Encourage all clients to wear hearing aids if they have them. Recommend that the hearing-impaired client be evaluated by an audiologist. Assist the client with checking hearing aid batteries weekly. Most batteries can be purchased at pharmacies. Store hearing aids in a safe place when not in use; they are small and can get lost easily. Proper hearing aid use and maintenance is critical. Too many times, hearing-impaired persons miss out or misunderstand simple conversations because they do not hear words correctly. The person can feel unnecessarily isolated; having properly working hearing aids is an easy solution.

More Information

National Institute on Deafness and other Communication Disorders
(presented by the National Institute of Health)
31 Center Drive, MSC 2320
Bethesda, MD 20892-2320
http://www.nidcd.nih.gov/
http://nihseniorhealth.gov/hearingloss/toc.html

Heart Disease

There are many types of heart disease, including angina, arrhythmia, artherosclerosis (hardening of the arteries), congestive heart failure, high blood pressure, stroke, and heart attack. Atherosclerosis occurs when plaque build-up causes the arteries to narrow, thereby limiting blood flow to the heart and brain. This can be a result of high blood pressure. When plaque breaks free from arterial walls, a blood clot can form, blocking the artery and causing a heart attack or stroke. Heart attacks happen when blood flow to the heart is blocked and the heart muscle begins to die. In heart failure, the heart continues to pump blood but not efficiently. The body does not get the blood and oxygen it needs. Congestive heart failure, high blood pressure, and stroke are discussed in more detail in respective sections.

Signs and Symptoms

Signs of heart disease will vary depending on the type of heart condition. Heart attacks may start slow, with mild pain or discomfort. Warning signs that a heart attack is happening are:

Pressure or pain in the center of the chest that lasts more than a few minutes or goes away and comes back

Pain or discomfort in one or both arms, back, neck, jaw, or stomach
Shortness of breath
Breaking into a cold sweat
Nausea or lightheadedness, in combination with other symptoms
See "Signs and Symptoms" of congestive heart failure, high blood pressure, and stroke in their respective sections.

Treatment

The American Heart Association warns that if one or more of these signs are experienced, seek immediate medical attention. Blood-thinning medications to prevent clotting may be prescribed routinely or help in a crisis situation. Prevention is the best key to avoid or reduce heart disease and related disorders and should be approached by lowering blood pressure, exercising regularly, eating a healthy diet, quitting smoking, reducing cholesterol and fats, and keeping educated about heart health and warning signs (American Heart Association, 2004b).

The Care Provider's Role and Responsibilities

General, day-to-day duties may be assisting the care recipient with errands and light chores around the home. Remind care recipients with heart conditions to physically exert only as much as they can tolerate and as instructed by a physician. A care provider may need to monitor care recipients' conditions and report changes. Care providers can offer information about heart disease to the care recipient, including adaptations to lifestyle such as smoking cessation programs, exercise routines, and how to create a healthy diet.

More Information

American Heart Association (National Center)
7272 Greenville Avenue
Dallas, TX 75231
800-242-8721
http://www.americanheart.org

High Blood Pressure (HBP/Hypertension)

Blood pressure is the pressure of blood pushing against blood vessel walls when the heart pumps. Every time the heart beats, it sends blood out into the arteries. When the heart is pumping, blood pressure is higher; inversely, the heart is at rest between beats and blood pressure is lower. This is measured by two numbers: systolic and diastolic, with the systolic number written above or before the diastolic number. The benchmark numbers used to determine if blood pressure is high or low are 120/80. The systolic number measures the heart at work, which we see here as 120, and the diastolic number, 80, measures the heart at rest. Blood pressure is considered high when the systolic is over 140 and the diastolic number is over 90 for an extended length of time.

High blood pressure contributes to strokes, heart attack or heart failure, and kidney failure.

Signs and Symptoms

Often, high blood pressure is not felt. Symptoms are silent and that is why monitoring blood pressure is very important, especially for people at risk. Factors for high risk include:

Family history of high blood pressure
African Americans
Age (people over 35)
Excess weight or obesity
Physical inactivity
High salt intake
High alcohol intake
Diabetes, gout, and kidney disease
Pregnancy
Women on birth control pills who are overweight, have HBP during pregnancy, have a family history of HBP, or have mild kidney disease

Treatment

The most common approach for treating high blood pressure is medication, usually a blood thinner to keep blood flowing. Regular or even daily blood pressure checks are strongly suggested by health care professionals. Physicians and health care professionals recommend lifestyle and behavioral changes to reduce stress, promote relaxation, and encourage healthy living habits through diet and exercise. Managing high blood pressure can prevent strokes or other cardiovascular conditions and it should be taken seriously. Persons with high blood pressure should work closely with a physician and other health care professionals to monitor, control, and prevent potential problems (American Heart Association, 2004a).

The Care Provider's Role and Responsibilities

As with other heart conditions, care providers may be asked to run errands and perform light home chores, or monitor that medication routines are being followed and report changes in care recipients' status as needed. Care providers should encourage a care recipient with high blood pressure to eat a healthy diet and follow an exercise regimen as suggested by a physician. Again, providing the care recipient with information and education about HBP, heart disease, and stroke is helpful.

More Information

American Heart Association
National Center

7272 Greenville Avenue
Dallas, TX 75231
800-242-8721
http://www.americanheart.org

Impaired and Loss of Vision

Visual impairment ranges from mild to severe. A person who uses any type of visual corrective device (eyeglasses, contact lenses, medicine, or surgery) will likely still have imperfect vision. Age contributes to many eye diseases and impairments. Age-related macular degeneration (AMD) is the leading cause of vision loss in older adults. Glaucoma, the leading cause of blindness in the United States, is the build-up of fluid pressure in the eye that ultimately damages the optic nerve. Also common to older adults are cataracts, which cause the gradual clouding of the eye lens of one or both eyes. Cataracts are not contagious and do not spread from one eye to the other. Often cataracts will occur with AMD or glaucoma.

Signs and Symptoms

The most notable symptom of macular degeneration is the deterioration of central vision that impairs the visual field even if peripheral vision is intact. Symptoms typical of cataracts are blurry vision, colors that seem faded, glare, not being able to see well at night, double vision, and frequent prescription changes of eyewear.

Treatment

Some conditions and diseases may be detected early with regular eye examinations. The symptoms, causes, severity, and stage of impairment determine the best treatment for diseases of the eye. Macular degeneration can be treated with medicines or surgery, though there is no cure. Glaucoma is usually treated with prescription eye drops or surgery or both. A new eyeglass prescription, brighter lighting, antiglare glasses, and magnifying lenses can help in the early stages of cataracts. Cataract surgery becomes an option when vision loss interferes with daily activities and functioning. The cloudy lens is removed from the eye and replaced with an artificial lens. There are different types of cataract surgeries and different procedures for each process. Optometrists and ophthalmologists (see "Physicians and Specialists" at the end of this chapter) are eye specialists who should be consulted for an evaluation to determine the best treatment approach.

The Care Provider's Role and Responsibilities

In addition to errands and home chores, care providers can assist visually impaired care recipients by suggesting and obtaining vision aids. Contact a local visual aid organization for service and product information. Recommend that the care recipient regularly visit an optometrist or ophthalmologist for regular eye examinations, current prescriptions, and suggestions for other visual aids and treatments.

Use a black marker when writing notes, messages, or calendar entries; most times, the contrast of black ink on white paper is easier to see. Care providers should make an effort to write clearly and legibly, to write large, and to use good penmanship. If a person's vision is severely impaired or blind, do not rearrange things around the house without first discussing with the care recipient; many visually impaired people keep things in the same place, knowing exactly where to find what they are looking for. Care providers may need to read mail and identify objects. For example, a visually impaired person may not be able to distinguish between a can of corn and a can of pineapple. The care provider may need to rearrange kitchen cupboards to store canned vegetables in one location and canned fruits in another. If the care recipient does not have the home or kitchen organized to meet this need, the care provider may suggest methods for organizing systems. Ask the visually impaired person how to best help. Everyone has varying routines and unique ways to accomplish routine tasks.

More Information

National Eye Institute
2020 Vision Place
Bethesda, MD 20892-3655
301-496-5248
http://www.nei.nih.gov

Kidney Disorder (Renal Disease)

Almost everyone has two kidneys located on either side of the spine, behind the abdomen and below the rib cage. The kidneys filter blood by removing waste and excess water through urine. Kidney disease results when the filtering agents, called nephrons, become damaged and unable to filter blood and remove waste.

Signs and Symptoms

There are no obvious symptoms of kidney disease in the early stages, and damage usually occurs over time. As the disease progresses, a person may experience:

Feeling weak and tired
A loss of appetite
Inability to sleep
Unable to think clearly
Swelling of the feet and ankles

Diabetes or problems with regulating blood sugar, high blood pressure, and hereditary traits (an immediate family member with kidney disease) are risk factors of kidney disease. A physician will measure proteins in the urine and creatinine in the blood to detect renal disease.

Treatment

Usually kidney disease is not cured but managed. A person with risk factors should consult with a physician for prevention and treatment plans. A person with diabetes needs to closely monitor and control blood-sugar levels. Blood pressure should be monitored and controlled through medications especially when kidney function is reduced. A kidney transplant or dialysis is used when kidneys fail completely. There are two types of dialysis treatments, hemodialysis and peritoneal dialysis, which have distinct differences and dietary needs. If your care recipient receives dialysis treatment, it is important to know which treatment and guidelines to follow. Irreversible kidney failure known as End Stage Renal Disease (ERSD) is usually life threatening.

The Care Provider's Role

There are no specific tasks a care provider should do for a person with a kidney disease. Monitoring health status, running errands, and performing home chores are likely needed. Discuss with care recipients their exact needs and determine routines and responsibilities based on individual needs and expectations.

More Information

National Kidney Disease Education Program
(presented by the National Institute of Diabetes and Digestive
    and Kidney Diseases, NIDDK)
Building 31, Room 9A06
31 Center Drive MSC 2560
Bethesda, MD 20892-2560
http://www2.niddk.nih.gov

Lung Disease

Lung disease is an umbrella term for any disorder that makes breathing difficult and prohibits the body from getting enough oxygen. Cells in the body need oxygen to work and grow; lungs absorb the oxygen into the bloodstream and expel carbon dioxide. Respiration rate, the measure of lung capacity, decreases in age. Lung capacity determines the amount of oxygen transferred from the lungs to the blood, which transports oxygen throughout the body. Common air pollutants that can impact or damage lung capacity are bacteria, viruses, tobacco smoke, chemicals, dust, and automobile exhaust.

Two specific lung diseases commonly found in older adults are discussed here.

Chronic Obstructive Pulmonary Disease (COPD) occurs when the airways become obstructed and oxygen flow is restricted. Less air gets in and less gets out. Air sacs also lose their elasticity and do not work productively. Cigarette smoking and inhaling pollutants contribute to lung disease. Bronchitis and emphysema are types of COPD.

Signs and Symptoms

COPD develops over time and it may take years before signs become obvious. Signs of COPD are coughing up mucus, shortness of breath, wheezing, and chest tightness. These symptoms should be accurately diagnosed by a physician.

Treatment

COPD cannot be cured, though symptoms can be managed. Quitting smoking or removing air pollutants are effective approaches to reduce the risk of COPD or to slow progression of the conditions. Treatments depend on the severity of the symptoms and individual needs. Exercise and breathing trainings may be recommended as a care recipient is able to tolerate. Medication and the use of oxygen may be used to relieve symptoms; in severe cases, surgery may be required.

Pneumonia is very common in people over the age of 65. Bacteria, viruses, and fungi enter into the lungs and may cause infection, resulting in pneumonia. Accidentally inhaling a liquid or chemical into the lungs can also cause pneumonia. There are several different types of pneumonia; knowing what type of pneumonia—bacterial or viral—is diagnosed will ultimately direct care and treatment.

Signs and Symptoms

Pneumonia symptoms can gradually or suddenly appear. Influenza symptoms are common: cough, fever, chills, nausea, weakness, and muscle ache. People with pneumonia have difficulty breathing demonstrated by a shortness of breath or rapid breathing; in severe cases, chills and chest pains can occur. A physician or health care professional will need to take a chest x-ray and perform blood tests for proper diagnosis and treatment.

Treatment

Antibiotics are regularly prescribed to treat pneumonia, though the best method depends on the cause of the infection. Preventive measures against pneumonia are keeping hands clean, not smoking, and wearing a mask in dirty areas to prevent pollutants from entering the lungs. Pneumococcal pneumonia is a vaccine for bacterial infections, and effective against pneumococcal pneumonia.

The Care Provider's Role

It is likely that responsibilities will be tasks that minimize physical activity for care recipients with lung conditions. The living environment should be kept clean. Because a person with pneumonia or COPD may have compromised immune functioning, caregivers who are sick (such as having a cold or flu) should not visit the care recipient. Care providers can offer information and education about air filters, smoking cessation programs, medical equipment, and supportive breathing devices.

More Information

The American Lung Association (National Headquarters)
61 Broadway, 6th Floor
New York, NY 10006
212-315-8700
http://www.lungsusa.org

Mental Health

Mental health refers to how we manage and cope with the highs and lows of daily life and difficult life events. A mental illness refers to a disruption in mood, thought, and behavior that interferes with our social and psychological functioning. Research indicates that brain dysfunction as it relates to mental illness is a consequence of heredity, biological, or environmental factors.

There are many types of mental health conditions. The mental disorders listed here are common to the aging population. *Anxiety disorder* is a persistent preoccupation with an unreasonable fear. Post-traumatic stress disorder (PTSD) is a type of anxiety disorder in which a person who has experienced a traumatic event feels afraid and helpless after the event. The person has difficulty coping with and accepting the trauma. Obsessive Compulsive Disorder (OCD) is another type of anxiety disorder, characterized by repetitive, upsetting thoughts called obsessions. A compulsion is the unsuccessful, repeated approach of eliminating that obsession. For example, an obsession may be the constant fear of another person stealing personal belongings (this is a common fear of residents in nursing homes; it is debatable whether this is an obsession or a reality) and a compulsion that addresses the obsession may be guarding personal belongings by never leaving the room or even constantly counting and keeping an inventory of belongings.

Signs and Symptoms

Signs of general anxiety can include worry, tension, irritability, trouble getting or staying asleep, nightmares, and the fear of leaving the home. Physical symptoms may include chest pains, headaches, and trembling. Because there are different types of anxiety disorders, it is important to involve a physician or mental health professional who can make an accurate diagnosis for proper treatment.

Treatments

Medications and therapies are often recommended for most of these mental health conditions. Older adults can improve or maintain good mental health by staying engaged in daily routines, being active in areas of interest, spending time with loved ones, and exercising. In older years, many problems become layered with additional complications that can be stressful and overwhelming; these issues should be addressed one at a time. A supportive environment contributes significantly to the well-being of any person, especially for older adults.

The Care Provider's Role and Responsibilities

The care provider should provide support and compassion, using active listening skills to understand care recipient concerns and needs. Care providers should create pleasant and engaging opportunities for care recipients that may divert focus from stressors and sources of frustration. A care provider should never assume more responsibility than he or she is capable of and should be aware of personal and professional boundaries. The care providers must realize they cannot fix the problem and are likely not trained to handle such complex situations. Medical or mental health professionals should be involved, especially if the care recipient is demonstrating severe symptoms.

More Information

American Society on Aging
833 Market Street
Suite 511
San Francisco, CA 94103
http://www.asaging.org/index.cfm

Osteoporosis

Osteoporosis is a disease often found in the aging body, and is more common to women than men, though anyone is susceptible. With this disease, the bones weaken enough that they become brittle and break easily. The hip, spine, ankles, and wrist bones are the most vulnerable to breakage.

Signs and Symptoms

There are no signs or symptoms of the disease; it usually goes unnoticed until a bone breaks. A curved spine, stooped posture, and back pain can indicate that the spine has been fractured several times. Two noteworthy risk factors are gender and age. Women are at higher risk than men for osteoporosis because female bones are smaller and deteriorate faster. Bones become thin and weak with age, making an older person more susceptible to osteoporosis. Other risk factors are having a family history of the disease, being a white or Asian woman, certain medications, and having low bone mass, called osteopenia. A bone density test is used to diagnose osteoporosis, which tests the bone strength and density.

Treatment

Prevention and preventing fractures is important because there is no cure for osteoporosis. A well-balanced diet with large amounts of calcium and vitamin D is strongly encouraged, as well as maintaining a regular exercise program. Keeping the environment clutter free in order to prevent falls is critical. Medications that slow bone loss are available. A bone density test is used to diagnose osteoporosis, which tests the bone strength and density.

The Care Provider's Role and Responsibilities

Care providers can make the living environment safer by removing clutter and rearranging furniture to designate clear paths for walking. Installing grab bars and handrails in prominent places can also help minimize the risk of falling. Care recipients with osteoporosis may need to be educated about diet to increase their intake of calcium and vitamin D. Encourage the care recipient to be as active as able and to follow any recommended exercise programs. As conditions worsen, the care recipient will probably need assistance with personal and household routines.

More Information

National Institute of Health, Senior Health
http://www.nihseniorhealth.gov/osteoporosis/toc.html

Pain

Pain management has become a standard medical practice to serve people suffering from chronic pain lasting 6 months or longer. Chronic pain can be a symptom of another disease or condition, such as arthritis, cancer, or diabetes, though many times people do not know the source of their pain. The constant sensation of pain or not feeling well can affect daily life and become wearing on the body and mind, causing depression and anger.

Signs and Symptoms

Pain is the signal a body sends to signify a problem. Pain is either treated and goes away or it is managed and becomes a way of life. There are different types of pain—sharp, dull, shooting, or achy. It can be constant or intermittent, and it may last a few days or a few years.

Treatment

It is important to tell the doctor everything about the pain, including the type and duration of pain, for proper treatment. Pain relievers, anti-inflammatory medicines, surgery, and even antidepressants are used to manage pain. For some chronic pain situations, physical therapy or other exercise may be recommended. Lifestyle changes and relaxation techniques have also been found effective for pain management.

The Care Provider's Role and Responsibilities

The role of the care provider is to make the care recipient comfortable. This may be through positioning or locating appropriate adaptive equipment or making blankets, food, and water readily accessible. It may simply be making sure items of comfort are accessible. Promoting relaxation can be very helpful to a care recipient in constant pain; be sure to learn what is comforting to the care recipient. Music may be soothing, or one-on-one conversation and sharing can be relaxing. The care provider should talk with the care recipient about the effectiveness of the pain management plan and monitor that the care recipient is taking medications as prescribed. Any changes in pain levels or indications that prescriptions are not being followed correctly—including suspicion of medication abuse—should be reported to supervisors or family members. Encourage the care recipient to keep a daily pain journal to record the time pain occurs, medications taken, discussions with doctors, and pain-management solutions.

More Information

Partners Against Pain
One Stamford Forum
Stamford, CT 06901-3431
888-726-7535
http://www.partnersagainstpain.com

Parkinson's Disease

Parkinson's disease is a neurological disorder that affects the nerve cells (neurons) in the brain that control movement. The chemical dopamine is produced by neurons that send signals to the body to coordinate movement. With Parkinson's, the dopamine-producing neurons are damaged or die. The National Institute of Neurological Disorders and Stroke (2007) reports that Parkinson's usually starts around the age of 60, though it can occur in people younger, and it is more common in men than women.

Scientists and researchers are still trying to determine the cause of this debilitating disease. At this time, genetic mutations are being linked to Parkinson's. Additionally, it is believed that environmental factors may play a part in developing the disease. Toxins may influence symptoms and progression of the disease, and viruses may possibly influence symptoms.

Signs and Symptoms

Symptoms occur gradually and may initially appear as a general slowing in speaking, moving, tiredness, or depression for no apparent reason. Symptoms usually start on one side of the body, eventually affecting both sides as the disease progresses. Characteristic signs that become more obvious can include:

Trembling of hands, arms, legs, jaw, and face
Rigidity and stiffness in the arms, legs, and trunk
Slow movement (called Bradykinesia)
Slow speech patterns
Unsteady balance, gait, and coordination
Flat affect (lacking facial expressions and liveliness)

As the disease progresses even further, other symptoms can be:
Bowel or bladder problems
Changes in speech and speaking
Dementia or other cognitive impairment
Depression
Difficulty with chewing and swallowing
Difficulty staying asleep, restless sleep, or nightmares
Fatigue/loss of energy
Muscle cramps
Pain
Sexual dysfunction
Skin problems (common for the skin on the face to become oily)
Sudden drop in blood pressure (orthostatic hypotension) when a person
stands up

The Hoehn and Yahr Scale is used to describe how Parkinson's symptoms progress (see Tip 5.2).

Tip 5.2

Hoehn and Yahr Scale

Stage one

Symptoms on one side of the body.

Stage two

Symptoms on both sides of the body. No balance impairment.

Stage three

Balance impairment. Mild to moderate disease; physically independent.

> **Stage four**
>
> Severe disability; still able to walk or stand unassisted.
>
> **Stage five**
>
> Wheelchair bound or bedridden, unless assisted.
>
> *From:* www.ninds.nih.gov/disorders/parkinsons_disease/detail_parkinsons_
> disease.htm#90633159

Treatment

Parkinson's symptoms are managed while conditions deteriorate over time. There is no cure. With early detection and appropriate treatment, many Parkinson's patients live a long time with the disease. Exercise and alternative therapies (i.e., yoga, tai chi, massage therapy) may help to keep the muscles and body flexible. Medications are the most common treatment and there are three categories. The first category is medications that increase dopamine levels in the brain. The second category treats motor symptoms to reduce tremors and muscle rigidity. The third category treats the nonmotor symptoms, such as depression, hallucinations, or delusions. Patients who do not have success with drug treatments may undergo surgical procedures.

The Care Provider's Role and Responsibilities

The care provider must be patient, flexible, and understanding. People with Parkinson's move slowly but should be encouraged to be as active as able. A care provider may plan light exercise and walking schedules during visits, or suggest other forms of physical activity. Duties may include assistance, supervision, and suggestions for simplifying daily routines.

The care provider may also act as a support to the family. Encourage family members to become educated about the disease to understand the physical, mental, and cognitive changes that can occur. Also, suggest that family attend local support group meetings; if needed, provide family members with meeting dates, times, and locations.

More Information

National Parkinson Foundation
1501 N.W. 9th Avenue
Bob Hope Road
Miami, FL 33136-1494
305-243-6666 or 800-327-4545
http://www.parkinson.org

Stroke (CVA/Cerebral Vascular Accident)

Strokes are a result of insufficient blood flow through the circulatory system where not enough oxygen reaches the brain. A stroke occurs when a blood vessel (artery) carrying oxygen and nutrients to the brain is narrowed, blocked, or burst. When this happens, the affected part of the brain does not get the blood carrying the oxygen it needs and it starts to die.

Signs and Symptoms

Common warning signs of stroke are sudden:

> Numbness or weakness of face, arm, or leg, especially on one side of the body
> Confusion, dizziness, and loss of balance or coordination
> Trouble speaking or understanding
> Vision problems in one or both eyes
> Trouble walking
> Severe headache with no known cause

The effects of a stroke depend on which part and how much of the brain has been affected. Remember, one side of the brain controls the opposite side of the body; if a stroke happens in the right part of the brain, the left side of the body will be affected.

Signs that a stroke occurred on the *right* side of the brain could be vision problems, paralysis on the left side of the body, and memory loss. Indicators that the stroke occurred in the *left* side of the brain could be paralysis on the right side of the body, speech and language problems, and memory loss.

Treatment

There are different types of treatments for strokes depending on the type of stroke and severity. Medications such as anticoagulants (blood thinners) are used to prevent a stroke, and other treatments may include surgery to remove blockages. Strokes occur with varying severity. A physician will make an appropriate diagnosis and a suitable treatment plan after performing a neurological examination, a CT scan, and multiple tests (American Heart Association, 2004a).

The Care Provider's Role and Responsibilities

The roles and responsibilities of the care provider will vary depending on the physical and cognitive abilities of the care recipient. Usually, responsibilities include assisting the care recipient with physical tasks that they may no longer be able to perform or that are too time-consuming for them. Chores around the home and errand running are typical tasks. This assistance with nonpersonal care routines may give the care recipient additional time to perform other measures of self-care, making it feasible for the care recipient to maintain an independent lifestyle. Additionally, care recipients may need information for improving their diet and support devices for managing daily routines more easily. For persons severely affected by a stroke, creating pleasant experiences through one-on-one attention is helpful.

More Information

American Stroke Association (National Center)
7272 Greenville Avenue
Dallas, TX 75231
888-478-7653
http://www.strokeassociation.org

Physicians and Specialists

Physicians regularly refer patients to specialists for a detailed examination of specific conditions, specialized tests, and diagnoses. Specialists commonly involved with the older population and their areas of expertise are listed here.

Anesthesiologist: disorders of the immune system

Audiologist: hearing defects and treatments

Cardiologist: problems with the cardiovascular system—heart, arteries, and veins

Colon and Rectal Surgeon: bowel, bladder, intestines, and digestive tract

Dentist: teeth and gums

Dermatologist: conditions of the skin, hair, and nails

Endocrinologist: disorders of glands and hormones

Gastroenterologist: disorders of the stomach, intestines, and digestive tract

Geriatrician: general medical conditions of the aging

Gerontologist: biological, psychological, and sociological issues of aging

Gynecologist: female reproductive system

Hematologist: diseases of the blood, bone marrow, and vascular system

Internist: prevention, diagnosis, and treatment of adult diseases

Nephrologist: treatment of kidney disorders

Neurologist: disorders affecting the nervous system

Oncologist: cancer treatments

Ophthalmologist: treatments and surgeries of eye problems

Optician: makes eyeglasses and lenses

Optometrist: disorders of the eye; makes prescriptions for lenses

Orthopedist: disorders of bone and connective tissue

Orthotist: mechanical devices and equipment that support bones and joints

Osteopath: manipulation of the skeleton, muscles, and tissues

Otolaryngologist: ear, nose, and throat disorders

Pharmacist: medication information and education

Podiatrist: problems of the feet

Psychiatrist: emotional and mental health disorders (and has the ability to prescribe medications)

Psychologist: psychological testing and counseling

Pulmonologist: problems with the lungs and respiratory system

Radiologist: x-rays and other pictures or tests that show the inside of the body

Rheumatologist: problems of the musculoskeletal system and joints

Urologist: disorders of the urinary tract

Tip 5.3

Statistics of Health and Chronic Conditions

Many older adults have at least one chronic condition, though many have multiple conditions. Among the most frequently occurring conditions of the aging population in 2003–2004:

Hypertension 52%

Diagnosed arthritis 50%

Heart disease 32%

Any cancer 21%

Diabetes 17%

Note: Information retrieved from the U.S. Department of Health and Human Services Administration on Aging Web site, http://www.aoa.gov/press/fact/pdf/ss_stat_profile.pdf

Summary

The conditions and diseases in this chapter are commonly seen in the aged population. (Statistics of common age-related diagnoses and conditions can be found in Tip 5.3.) It does not mean all of these illnesses will occur with age, nor does it mean that the diseases cannot occur in younger populations. Care providers should be aware of and prepare for these age-related conditions. To learn more, contact related local chapters or national organizations for condition- and disease-specific information. Care providers can provide personal, quality care when they are educated about the conditions, causes, signs and symptoms, and treatments of diseases. The role of the care provider is to offer support and to act as a sounding board while the care recipient processes options to make decisions, not to recommend medical advice.

Questions

Why is it important for care providers to have basic understandings of age-related conditions and diseases?

What should care providers do when they observe changes in care recipient symptoms?

What important functions does a care provider serve to ailing care recipients?

Summary Tips

Be very clear on care recipient and family expectations of duties and responsibilities as it relates to a care recipient's disease process.

Seek medical advice and attention when there are significant changes in a care recipient's health care status.

Contact local chapters or national headquarters for disease-specific information to learn more about conditions, symptoms, and possible treatments.

Share information with care recipients and family members as it relates to the circumstances; encourage all involved to learn more and attend support groups as needed.

Helpful Web Sites

Medline Plus: U.S. National Library of Medicine and the National Institute of Health resource base of health-related information at http://www.nlm.nih.gov/medlineplus/healthtopics.html

American Heart Association: http://www.americanheart.org

American Psychological Association: http://www.apa.org

National Institute of Health, Senior Health: http://nihseniorhealth.gov/listoftopics.html

Suggested Reading

Anderson, Mary Ann. (2007). *Caring for older adults holistically* (4th ed.). Philadelphia: Davis, F. A. Practical and positive approach to working with the aging population, emphasizing health-promoting lifestyles.

Mace, Nancy, & Rabins, Peter. (2006). *The 36-hour day: A family guide to caring for persons with Alzheimer's disease, related dementing illnesses, and memory loss in later life.* Baltimore, MD: John Hopkins University Press. Informational resource and guidebook for caregivers of persons with Alzheimer's disease and other dementias.

The Terminally Ill Client

6

In This Chapter, You Will Learn

1. What it means to have a terminal diagnosis

2. Stages of grief

3. Emotional and physical changes during the dying process

4. The signs of active dying

5. The role of hospice care

Why This Matters

Working with the terminally ill is a paradoxical experience: It can present challenging emotional, mental, and physical responsibilities while providing the most rewarding gifts of what life has to offer. The subjects of death and dying are difficult for U.S. society; death and dying are not discussed at the dinner table, the coffee shop, or around the water cooler at work. Fortunately, the hospice movement is bringing awareness to the concept of dying with dignity and attention to the care choices for a dying person. The terminally ill have changing emotional and physical needs. Home care providers and caregivers should know what to expect during the dying process and be prepared to meet those needs through measures of comfort and supportive care. Caring for the terminally ill teaches not only about dying, but more about living.

A Terminal Diagnosis

Doctors may diagnose a person with a terminal illness when they see a continual and consistent downward spiral in a person's health and ability to function. To be terminal means that there is no cure and death will inevitably result. A person may live with a disease for a long period of time although the doctor does not consider it life threatening until the end stages. This is different from a chronic condition in which a person has persistent and long-lasting circumstances. Arthritis and diabetes are good examples of chronic conditions, although diabetes can become terminal when symptoms can longer be treated and only managed. A person with Alzheimer's or heart disease will not be considered terminal until the doctor determines the disease has progressed to the end stages, when the direction of the disease cannot be reversed. Other terminal illness diagnosis can include cancer, emphysema, liver and kidney failure, heart disease, and AIDS. A terminal diagnosis means that the doctor does not usually expect a person to live beyond 12 months, though a person typically has a diagnosis of 6 months or less to live to be eligible for hospice care. However, no one ever knows for certain.

The dying process encompasses the emotional, spiritual, and physical changes that are experienced when a person is diagnosed with a terminal illness or when death becomes imminent. According to hospice practices, a good death can occur when there is an absence of emotional, spiritual, and physical pain. A terminally ill person is more capable of resolving emotional and spiritual discomfort when pain is managed. The terminally ill person is encouraged to reflect on life, review relationships, and take part in end-of-life and funeral planning. The dying person should participate only as able and to the extent that personal comfort allows, as it can be emotionally difficult for some to make their own funeral arrangements. The body will experience various physical and physiological changes throughout the dying process depending on the person's disease and its progression. To offer quality care, any home care provider and caregiver needs to expect these changes and prepare to provide the client with enduring support.

Emotional Stages

Elisabeth Kubler-Ross, medical doctor and psychiatrist, is internationally known for her expertise with the dying process. Dr. Kubler-Ross has done extensive work and research with people at the end of their life and has identified five stages of emotions a dying person and family may experience during the process: denial, anger, bargaining, depression, and acceptance. Though not every person will experience all five emotions or in the order Dr. Kubler-Ross suggests, her Five Stages of Grief model is widely known and accepted for those coping with grief or death (see Tip 6.1).

Emotional needs will vary for each person as they move through these five stages and the dying process, though there are common sensitivities and wishes. A general feeling of fear is frequently heard from terminally ill patients. It is imperative that the person feels safe with the care that is being provided. A piece of this security is reassuring the dying person that his or her feelings are normal; providing the dying person with opportunities to share feelings and concerns with a trusted other is very important as is allowing the person the chance to see family and friends and to talk about the past.

Tip 6.1

The Five Stages of Grief

Denial: does not believe the circumstances
A person may say, "It's not true" or "It is not happening to me."
Anger: resentment of the situation
A person may say, "The doctors do not know what they're doing" or "Why me?"
Bargaining: making deals with their God to live longer
A person may say, "Let me live to see my daughter get married" or "I'll go to church every day if I can live longer."
Depression: a sense of loss and sadness
A person may say, "Why should I do anything?" or "I cannot fight any longer."
Acceptance: admits the circumstances and makes appropriate preparations
A person may say, "It will be ok" or "I am ready to make funeral arrangements."

Note: Copyright 1969, from *On Death and Dying* by Elisabeth Kubler-Ross.

Physical Changes

Disease processes are different and will physically and emotionally affect each body differently. Various symptoms will be observed through the progression and stages of a terminal illness. A caregiver may see symptoms common to the dying process, though they do not necessarily mean that a person is in the active stage of dying. These signs could be a failure to thrive (physically or emotionally), increased periods of sleep, weakness, significant weight loss, and a decrease in food and fluid intake. These symptoms could indicate that a person's body is shutting down. Symptoms should be evaluated by a medical professional, who is better trained to determine the stage of the disease. During active dying, call the physician or members of the hospice team when the following changes are observed:

Level of consciousness
Skin color (paleness or mottling)
Increased swelling
Deep, shallow, irregular, or other abnormal breathing
Unresponsive to touch or pain
Very low blood pressure

A dying person may feel clammy and cold to the touch because blood is not circulating to certain parts of the body; this usually occurs first in the hands, arms, feet, and legs. A person may start to mottle, which is when the skin changes to a bluish-purple color, also known as cyanosis or being cyanotic, when circulation stops in the extremities.

A care recipient can be at home or in an assisted living facility, hospital, or nursing home during these final stages or when actively dying; in any environment, calm and quiet surroundings are typically preferred. Home care providers and other caregivers should make all attempts to keep the terminally ill person comfortable. If the person was diagnosed with a terminal illness before reaching the end stage of a disease, it is likely that arrangements for hospice have been made, which will provide additional care and services to support the care recipient and family.

Hospice Care

Hospice is special care for the dying that focuses on pain management that does not treat or cure a disease. Hospice does not promote life-extending measures. The purpose of hospice is to provide dignity of life and death through comfort care, known as *palliative care*. Hospice efforts create comfort and quality of life in the dying process for the terminally ill, family members, and significant others.

Care providers offer in-the-moment emotional support to the dying as well as family members. Care providers who work with the terminally ill should be prepared for unpredictable care situations and must have the ability to adjust to changing circumstances. A person providing care to the dying must accept various lifestyles shaped by socioeconomic status, race, and religion. Personality and conditions of mental health also affect the way in which hospice care is delivered and received. A keen sense of the dying person's needs can influence and build upon the hospice caregiving situation.

What Does It Mean for a Person Who Receives Hospice Care?

In order for a person to receive hospice care, he or she will have a prognosis of less than 6 months to live, a Do Not Resuscitate Order (DNR), and the doctor's consent to receive comfort care, not treatment. Hospice care includes medical, nursing, and personal care aide services, and may include brief hospitalizations and respiratory treatments to make breathing less difficult. Comfort will be promoted by managing symptoms that create discomfort. The services of hospice are coordinated by a team that includes a medical doctor, nurse, pharmacist, social worker, clergy person, and personal care aide. Additionally, ancillary team members may include professionals from alternative therapies—for example, a massage therapist. Team members' roles have specific responsibilities that contribute to the individualized care of the terminally ill person, family, and significant others. The multidisciplinary hospice team provides support and education of the dying process, they do not tell a person how to die. Hospice workers listen and ask relevant questions that will lead the patient or family members to finding answers to personal questions. Hospice care services can include but are not limited to

Pain management
Direction with options of care
Arranging for medical equipment
Receiving medications
Respite and companion care
Assistance with transportation to doctor appointments
Guidance with funeral planning
Emotional support
Spiritual/clergy support
Grief counseling
Referrals for legal and financial issues

Who Pays for Hospice Care?

A hospice benefit program is provided through Medicare Part A that covers most costs under specific criterion, such as that the hospice agency providing care must be approved by Medicare to receive reimbursement. Medicare Part A (Centers for Medicare and Medicaid Services, 2007b) will pay for hospice care for the person who

Is eligible for Medicare Part A
Is diagnosed with a terminal illness with a prognosis of less than 6 months to live
Is receiving care from a Medicare-approved hospice agency
Elects the hospice benefit, waiving rights to Medicare payments for services not related to the terminal illness

Medicare pays for services associated only with the terminal illness and related conditions, which may include (Centers for Medicare and Medicaid Services, 2007b):

Doctor and nursing care
Related medical equipment and supplies
Pain management medications
Home health aid and homemaker services
Physical, occupational, and speech therapy
Dietary counseling
Clergy services
Medical social services
Bereavement counseling
Short-term hospitalizations and respite care
Other medically necessary and reasonable services determined by the care team

Medicare does not pay for treatments to cure the terminal illness or for treatments that are not considered medically reasonable or necessary. A care provider that is not arranged through the hospice team or care that could be received from the elected hospice but is provided by another will not be paid for by Medicare. Services that are not considered medically reasonable and necessary are also not covered by Medicare. Hospice benefits through Medicare have very specific guidelines for eligibility and payment availability. Home care recipients and their families who are considering hospice services should be directed to nurses, social workers, or case managers for accurate information of Medicare's role in paying for hospice care.

Summary

The goal when caring for the terminally ill patient is to manage pain: Home care providers and other caregivers should make all attempts to keep the dying person comfortable. Dr. Elisabeth Kubler-Ross has identified five emotional stages a dying person may experience, which is well-known as the Five Stages of Grief: denial, anger, bargaining, depression, and acceptance. The stages of grieving and the dying process are intimate; no two people will have the same experience. The terminally ill and dying person will also experience physical changes throughout the disease process and in the end stages of life that may include:

No food or fluid intake
Diminishing level of consciousness
No response to physical or verbal stimulation
Irregular and labored breathing through the mouth
Incontinence or significant decrease in urine or bowel output

Hospice is special care for the dying and family members. The goal of hospice is to manage symptoms, especially pain, and not to seek treatments to cure disease or terminal illness. Hospice care includes services from a doctor, nurse, personal care aides, and clergy, as well as bereavement counseling, medical social services, dietary counseling, physical or occupational therapies, pain management medications, and medical equipment and supplies. Medicare pays for hospice benefits when the care recipient with a terminal illness diagnosis has a prognosis of less than 6 months to live, waives the rights of Medicare payments for services not related to the terminal illness, is determined eligible for Medicare Part A, and is receiving services from a Medicare-approved hospice agency. Home care providers should direct care recipients and family members to appropriate resources, such as a nurse or social worker, for complete and accurate information about hospice and the Medicare hospice benefits plan.

Questions

What is the difference between a terminal illness and chronic condition?
Alzheimer's disease is a terminal illness. True or False?
Name the Five Stages of Grief as identified by Elisabeth Kubler-Ross.
What comments may be heard as a terminally ill person moves through each phase of the dying process?

What is an important opportunity home care providers should provide the hospice patient?

What are three physical changes a person in the end stages of life may experience?

What are signs that a person is actively dying?

Are hospice services available in a long-term-care environment?

What are the three eligibility criteria for a person to enroll in hospice?

Hospice is known for seeking aggressive treatments to restore a person's health. True or False?

Who does hospice help?

Summary Tips

Place phone numbers of hospice team members within easy reach for all caregivers.

Provide a calm, quiet, and peaceful environment.

Refer the physician, nurse, or social worker to a client or family who is considering hospice care.

Helpful Web Sites

Hospice Foundation of America: provides information to help people personally and professionally cope with terminal illness, death, grief, and bereavement at http://www.hospicefoundation.org

National Hospice Foundation: offers consumer and caregiver services, professional leadership, research, legislative advocacy, communications, international development, and issues related to quality care at the end of life at http://www.nationalhospicefoundation.org

National Hospice and Palliative Care Organization: offers education and resources for those dealing with end-of-life care at http://www.nhpco.org/templates/1/homepage.cfm

Suggested Reading

Baird, Robert, & Rosenbaum, Stuart. (2003). *Caring for the dying*. Amherst, NY: Prometheus Books. The role of hospice and palliative care, spiritual needs of the dying and the caregiver's role, and legal and end-of-life issues.

Beresford, Larry. (1993). *The hospice handbook*. Boston: Little, Brown. Complete guide to choosing hospice care.

Coberly, Margaret. (2002). *Sacred passage: How to provide fearless, compassionate care for the dying*. Boston: Shambhala. Practical advice on the physical, emotional, and spiritual dimensions of caring for the dying.

Kubler-Ross, Elisabeth. (1997). *On death and dying* (1st ed.). New York: Scribner Classics. How death affects the patient and the professionals who care for them, through samples and interviews. Dr. Kubler-Ross introduces her model of the Five Stages of Grief.

Caring for Couples

7

In This Chapter, You Will Learn

1. Situations of partner care

2. To identify emotions of partners in care

3. Defining couples

4. Respite care

Why This Matters

As services are being delivered to more people in their homes or alternative living arrangements, home health care providers are seeing an increased trend of caring for more than one recipient at a time. The advantage to caring for more than one person is that services can be all encompassing to members of one household. Simultaneously providing care to more than one recipient requires a careful, structured balance of completing tasks while tending to emotional responses from each partner. Conflicts in personalities and how care routines are expected to be delivered not only occur with the care recipient but can occur with the care partner as well, especially under complicated circumstances. If only one person in the living arrangement is receiving care, home care providers typically consult with the partner-in-care to set up services such as meal planning, scheduling appointments, arranging transportation, and other incidentals. Care providers who build relationships with care partners can offer quality services through teamwork that will benefit the home care situation.

Caring for Couples

Historically, it has been common for women to provide care to husbands, fathers, sons and brothers; in the 21st century, more and more men are becoming caregivers for wives, mothers, sisters, and daughters. Because men and women are living longer, there are more people dealing with care issues that present diverse situations of caregiving.

Regardless of gender, there is only so much one person can do while maintaining a household and managing health issues for oneself and another at the same time. Caregiving is challenging for able-bodied adults and it is more challenging for people with compromised functioning who need to balance the physical and emotional demands of a caregiving situation. As the inclusion of home health services are the preferred alternative to facility placement, providing home care to couples or partners is occurring more frequently.

Situations of Partner Care

The most typical home care situation is where a care provider is employed to assist one care recipient. The roles and responsibilities of formal home care providers are influenced by the involvement of informal and family caregivers. It is also common that formal care providers are employed to give assistance and oversee care to more than one person in the home. Care providers who are hired to assist only one care recipient though realistically end up overseeing the care of an additional person in the home, while less expected, does regularly occur. This situation becomes complicated when the partner, for whom assistance is not arranged, does not easily accept necessary assistance from a care provider who must then divide efforts within the determined time frame. This delicate situation can hinder the care provided to the initial care recipient.

Care providers assist caregiving situations of more than one person by

Understanding emotional and physical needs of the care recipient
Understanding emotional and physical needs of the care partner
Creating balance between the needs of each
Establishing well-organized household systems and routines
Arranging additional service provisions

Emotions of Partners in Care

Exclusive dynamics are presented in caregiving situations involving partners that are missing when working with individuals. Real or perceived inadequacy of giving care is frequently expressed. Most people have little experience as a caregiver until the need arises; when it does, many feel incompetent in the new situation. Care partners may require more emotional support to manage the caregiving situation than the care recipient. It is very common for caregivers to predecease the care-recipient partner. The struggle for power is a relationship dynamic that can occur between a care partner (who is not receiving care) and the care provider. The suggestion of hiring formal caregivers may threaten the care partner. To justify real or perceived feelings of inadequacy, the care partner may routinely criticize formal care providers and insist that care is given in a particular manner. This may be a coping method to maintain control of the circumstances. Care providers are often in the position of balancing the needs of the care recipient with the needs of the care partner. It is reasonable to consider the impact, if any, a care partner or others will have on the home care recipient's needs and services.

The emotions of caring for a spouse, child, or significant other are typically different from the feelings of adult children who are caring for aging parents. While this can still be emotionally difficult, adults caring for aging parents expect this scenario because of natural, chronological order. Parents who provide care to a child because of disability or disease are presented with other emotional challenges because these situations of caregiving seem unnatural and out of order. Caregiving parents may feel responsible for the condition or experience feelings of guilt, often heard as "I wish this would have happened to me" and usually arrange and oversee ongoing services to meet their child's physical and emotional needs.

How the care partner copes with changing life circumstances as the result of the care recipient's medical condition or illness can lead to frustration and anger. Spousal or partner caregivers can become frustrated with the care recipient for becoming ill, especially if disruptive behaviors are evident. Care partners of those with Alzheimer's disease or other dementia usually become saddened and frustrated with the afflicted partner. Inappropriate behaviors can be difficult to manage and require constant supervision, which is physically tiring for the care partner, and it is emotionally difficult to observe the decline of a loved one. A care partner may mentally understand that the inappropriate behaviors are unintentional and symptoms of the disease though it is common

Case Study

Marie's fall resulted in a broken hip. After a hospitalization, she underwent therapy in a rehabilitation center for several weeks before she returned home to live with her husband, Paul. Marie learned to ambulate with a walker, which she continued to use and relied upon for safety when she returned home. She moved slowly and was cautious about her mobility. Personal care and household routines took more time to complete than prior to her fall. Bathing, dressing, and eating consumed most of her morning which left only a few hours in the afternoon for grocery shopping, running other errands, and going to doctors' appointments. Paul and Marie's daughter insisted that her parents seek formal assistance to help Marie with meal planning, errand running, and home organization tasks. Marie had always taken care of these responsibilities because Paul worked outside of the home, and even in his older years he continued to work in an office 5 days a week.

Diane was hired to provide these IADL services. As the care provider for Marie, Diane took her to the grocery store and assisted with the shopping. Diane made other shopping trips with a list that Marie provided when she did not feel well enough to leave the home. Once a week, Diane took Marie to the doctor's office. Diane's assistance with time-demanding household routines provided Marie the time she needed to recuperate. Additionally, Diane's services meant that Paul did not have to take time off of work to transport Marie to the doctor or shop and run errands.

As the benefits of Diane's service became more apparent, Paul began asking Marie and Diane to pick up his dry cleaning, visit the bank for him, and drive him to and from work. Diane's visits were scheduled for 2 hours a day, twice a week. This was just enough time for her to complete Marie's tasks; she did not have enough time to achieve Paul's extra requests. Paul and Marie did not want to hire Diane for additional hours. Instead, Diane divided the allotted time between tasks for Paul and Marie. As a result, some of Marie's household routines and responsibilities were not finished.

Paul offered more help around the house to accommodate what Marie was unable to perform. He became tired, short tempered, and resentful that Marie could not do more, and would often yell at her. His feelings and actions toward Marie complicated the situation. In trying to help Marie, he also had a fall and broke two rib bones. Paul's daughter arranged for him to have a home health care aide to assist him with personal care routines.

Diane continued to assist Marie with IADLs while Paul had another care provider who helped him primarily with ADLs and occasional IADLs. The additional service provisions for Paul allowed Diane to focus on Marie. They had time to run necessary errands and complete household routines, which permitted Marie the time she needed for rest and personal routines. Together, they could accomplish tasks to create a successful home caregiving situation for Paul and Marie.

for care partners to lose focus and become angry at the afflicted person rather than the disease. As a result, many care partners express anger at themselves for becoming upset at the afflicted partner who is unable to control inappropriate behaviors. Knowingly or not, the care-receiving partner may sense that the care partner is overwhelmed, which causes the care recipient to feel guilty or responsible for creating a perceived difficult situation. Unfortunately, both partners share feelings of guilt, anger, and frustration toward the other—for different reasons—while at the same time turn those feelings back on the self. It is a familiar, cyclical scenario between caregiving partners.

Defining Couples

It is important to define a couple because it is not just a husband and wife. When we think of a couple, it is immediately assumed that there is an intimate attachment though the relationships may be platonic. A couple can be an un-married man and woman who live together as well as two men or two women living together. A couple may be two people who only share living space. Home sharing with family members or nonfamily relations is a common living ar-rangement, especially in caregiving situations. Sisters, or sisters and brothers, often reunite in older years to take care of one another and share resources. A parent and adult child may live together because of financial constraints and physical or mental health conditions. Or simply, an adult child lives with an aging parent to benefit a caregiving situation. Other relationships in shared living places may be a grandchild with a grandparent, or nieces or nephews with aunts or uncles. They can be friends living together to make the best use of their combined resources.

A care recipient with a partner caring for more than one person in a home can be an ideal situation. Partners support each other by offering reminders and monitoring for problems when other care providers are not in the home. In healthy relationships, partners provide camaraderie and positive social in-teraction. If only one person is receiving assistance, the care partner can give formal care providers helpful hints and background information that will im-prove service delivery. Care providers and caring partners who work together will create a comprehensive care environment in the home, benefiting both the care recipient and partner.

Respite Care

Caregiving situations for couples and partners differ depending on personali-ties, perceived gender roles, health concerns, the physical environment, and the functional abilities of each partner. Necessary services range in responsibility and may fluctuate over time. Many couples and partners take advantage of re-spite care, which provides the primary caregiver relief away from the caregiv-ing situation. The goal of respite care is certainly to understand and meet the specific needs of the care recipient, though the *emphasis* of respite care is to provide relief services to the primary or other informal caregivers.

Respite care takes on various forms; it can be the provision of one-on-one attention in the home or taking the care recipient out of the home on errands and outings for stimulation. Household chores and home repair services are other areas of needed assistance, which is typical if the current care recipient previously performed the given task. As with individuals, couples or partners may need transportation to and from appointments or for other errand run-ning. Many service provisions for couples or partners are similar to those of individuals, though it may require simultaneous service provision to more than one person.

Summary

With longer life spans and more care services being delivered into the home, sit-uations of caring for couples are occurring with more frequency. The demands on men and women, who are acting as caregivers in later years, can increase the need for a variety of professional home care services. Caring for two people does not necessarily mean caring for a husband and wife or unmarried pair. Couples take various forms: parent-child or grandparent-grandchild, and relationships between two men or two women. Care providers may provide care for one or both partners. Either situation can present challenges unlike those when working with individuals without partners. Partners in caregiving situations often experience feelings of guilt and frustration; in many situations, anger cycles between the caring partner and the partner receiving care. The caring partner can become angry with the receiving partner and then becomes angry with the self. Relationship histories, gender roles, living environs, and health issues can affect how care is structured and delivered. Partners in care with care providers can work together to create a successful caregiving situation.

Questions

What complications can arise when working with couples or care partners?
How does a care partner benefit a caregiving situation?
Why does a caregiving partner experience guilt?
What is the cycle of anger that can occur between caregiving partners?
How does respite care benefit the care partner? The care recipient?

Summary Tips

Understand the care provider's roles and responsibilities, being aware that service provisions can change over time. Be flexible.
Be clear on who is receiving care.
Be sensitive to the emotions of both partners and the demands of caregiving.
Work as a team with spousal and family caregivers.

Helpful Web Sites

Information about caregiving issues and relationships: http://www.revolutionhealth.com
Issues related to spousal caregiving: http://www.caregiving.com
Effects of family caregiving: http://www.aamft.org

Suggested Reading

Lang, Frieder, & Fingerman, Karen. (2003). *Growing together: Personal relationships across the life span.* New York: Cambridge University Press. A look at personal relationships from childhood to later adulthood.

Martz, Sandra Haldeman. (2006). *Grow old along with me, the best is yet to be.* Kingston, RI: Moyer Bell. Stories and poems for men and women about daily aging, widowhood, and changing life roles.

Silverstone, Barbara. (1992). *Growing older together.* New York: Knopf Publishing Group. Accepting aging, changing family relationships, facing illness, coping with disability and death, and other issues facing couples over age 55.

About Activities

8

In This Chapter, You Will Learn

1. How activities add to quality of life

2. The difference between active and passive participation

3. About activities of life and activities of recreation

4. To recognize the companion's role in activity planning

5. How to choose effective and productive activities

Why This Matters

People feel better about themselves when they are productive: Accomplishing even simple tasks allows one to feel useful, which adds quality to life. Purposeful activities provide opportunities for feeling positive about the self. In older years, opportunities for productivity can become limited because it takes time and effort to find meaningful activity. An older adult may not have the physical or mental energy to look for purposeful, recreational activities when getting dressed can take an hour and health concerns are overwhelming. Even active older adults may not know how or where to find recreational activities that provide productive and purposeful results. Home care providers are hired to give quality care, which includes contributing to quality of life through purposeful and meaningful activity. It is a home care provider's responsibility to present a client with practical and recreational activity ideas that add value and purpose to each day.

Doing Things

Our days are filled with activities. Have you ever thought about all the activities you complete in one day? Can you think of a day when you did not have anything you had or wanted to do? Think about a typical day of work. Let's assume when you awoke you bathed and dressed, applied makeup, and styled your hair. The next activity is breakfast, which requires planning, preparing and eating, and then doing the dishes. On the way to work, books are returned at the library and a stop for gasoline is needed. The next 8 hours of work are filled with tasks (think of all the things you do on the job) and the day is not over. A visit to the grocery store on the way home is necessary, where you have to decide what foods to purchase. At home, you prepare meatloaf and salad for dinner. After eating, you exercise by taking a 20-minute walk. You water the garden, and finally sit down in front of the television to watch a favorite program. You go to bed, but before falling asleep, you decide the next chapter of the novel must be read so you can start the next book. A busy day of purposeful, practical, and recreational activities!

The types of activity we engage in change throughout life. Retirement activities replace the 40-hour workweek. Personal interests at age 70 may be significantly different than those at age 30. The ability to function influences activity involvement; for example, physical limitations may necessitate walking rather than riding a bicycle. A cognitively impaired person may decide to watch television or listen to music at home rather than attend social clubs and events. How an individual chooses to meet activity and productivity needs may be manifested differently in advanced age, yet the need does not necessarily cease.

Do not mistake doing nothing for relaxing! Many people consciously choose to do nothing as a form of relaxation while others are relaxed when painting, singing, or even dancing. It is acceptable for a care recipient to do nothing periodically or even routinely, for example, taking a nap every afternoon between 4:00 and 6:00 p.m. Care providers should evaluate the home care situation when a care recipient seldom or never wants to do *anything*—neither a practical nor recreational activity. A care recipient's lack of interest in participating in life events or routines can be signs of boredom, withdrawal, and isolation, which can lead to anxiety and depression. The more interested and active a care recipient is with life, the more connected he or she will feel to the self and others, which can decrease negative thought preoccupations and behaviors to promote positive actions and behaviors. It is not easy for a person to do nothing after 50 or more years of living a productive life. Physical, cognitive, and social stimulation aid a care recipient in healthy functioning during the aging process.

Activities and Quality of Life

Activities are opportunities to add meaning and satisfaction that contribute to quality of life. Activities alleviate boredom and fill a sense of purpose; when activities are useful, they improve our self-esteem and sense of self-worth. Intended or unintended outcomes are inevitable when we are actively involved, and passive participation will provide mental and social stimulation.

The ultimate goal of an activity is to add quality to life. In companion-care situations, the intended result of organized activities is to provide the client with a sense of personal meaning and value. Organized activities improve and maintain certain skills necessary to perform activities of daily life and the benefit is making use of these skills to improve quality of life. What are the skills used and the benefits of an activity?

Cognitive: decision-making skills, judgment, and the ability to remember or reminisce
Physical: fine and gross motor skills
Sensory: ability to perceive and use the five senses (seeing, hearing, smelling, tasting, and touching)
Social: communication and verbal skills, interacting with others, appropriate behaviors

Exercising cognitive, physical, sensory, and social skills is critical to both the higher functioning and cognitively impaired client. The use of these skills generates a sense of normalcy for the higher functioning client because it encourages autonomy, the act of governing the self. This instills confidence in individuals who may be lacking self-reliance after a distressing event. (For example, after a fall results in a broken hip, many older adults are hesitant and fearful of walking. The more they exercise their physical skills, the more confidence they will gain when it comes to walking and movement.) The stimulation of these skills promotes feelings of familiarity to thoughts and actions previously experienced in life for cognitively impaired care recipients. To achieve our purpose as caregivers and to help our care recipients achieve their maximum benefits, daily tasks and routines should be maximized to stimulate each skill—more than one at a time as able—while unoccupied time should be filled with fruitful activity. Table 8.1 applies goals, purposes, and action steps in a sample action plan for engaging others in activities. This tool is intended for use by the care provider, not the care receiver, as a guideline of what, why, and how to offer purposeful activity to care recipients. Activities can be structured or spontaneous, though having the goal, purpose, and action steps outlined can produce results quickly and efficiently.

Activities add quality to life when they are purposeful or practical and enjoyable to the care recipient. Effective activities are all-inclusive; use creativity to incorporate cognitive, physical, sensory, and social skills into activities. Integrating all five senses into one activity may not be possible or sensible—too much stimulation can be overwhelming to some care recipients. Be aware of the care recipient's moods, behaviors, and attitudes toward the activities you create.

It is easy to think that any activity is productive because it fills otherwise empty time. This is not always the case. An activity that merely passes time can sometimes lead to unintended consequences. Virginia, with slight cognitive impairment, was living in an assisted living facility. The Tuesday morning craft activity was to string beads, which she refused to do. She very vocally expressed

8.1	Example of an Activity Action Plan

Goal	Purpose	Action steps
To add quality of life in client's current situation	To improve or maintain: ♦ Cognitive functioning ♦ Social interactions ♦ Sensory perceptions ♦ Verbal/communication skills ♦ Physical activity To stimulate sensory perception	Provide opportunities for: a) Word games, puzzles, crosswords b) Outings to the grocery store, zoo, library, and park c) Exercise routines, walking, and ball toss d) Preparing noontime meal

her offense at the suggestion that she should participate in what she called a "dementia activity." Virginia believed she was capable of more productivity and was extremely insulted with the insinuation that she was not competent to perform at a higher level; she felt unchallenged, which lowered her self-esteem. This activity filled time, but it was not suitable for her. If a participant feels unchallenged or is unable to participate, the activity will not be successful.

Living environments and geographical locations influence how activities are conducted. The activity suggestions in this chapter may need to be adapted to meet available offerings, constraints, and the abilities of the care recipient. Their physical endurance may prohibit certain outings. Accessibility and transportation services are critical issues because neither is always available. Urban areas may not have a grocery store; substitute the outing with a visit to the "corner market." Parks and green spaces may not be nearby; if nature is of interest to the care recipient, bring the natural world to the care recipient with home videos, pictures, or live animals. Care recipients who live in apartment buildings may not have the option of a garden; use potted plants as an alternative. A rural or suburban community may not have an art museum; rather than travel to a larger city with this facility, consider visiting a local art gallery, shop, or other museum that is specific to the immediate area. Be creative and resourceful; use available, local resources to encourage sensory stimulation.

Active and Passive Participation

Care recipients' activity involvement is measured by active or passive participation. Active participation is when a participant puts forth effort and interest to be mentally, emotionally, or physically engaged in an activity. Passive participation is activity through sensory stimulation. Listening to the radio is a passive activity; dancing to music on the radio is active participation. The care recipient who goes to the library to look through magazines and check out books or the care recipient who is physically unable to go to the grocery store but creates the shopping list and cuts coupons are both engaged in active participation. Active participation should be encouraged for full advantages of stimulation, but do not discount the benefits of passive participation.

Some care recipients may only be able to participate passively due to cognitive or physical limitations. Passive participation can still provide sensory stimulation and social interaction. For example, a care recipient who is physically or cognitively unable to play a game of golf may enjoy time at the golf course or driving range. Or, the care recipient who is unable to assist with food preparation can interact with the care provider who is baking cookies by watching the process, smelling the results, and tasting the dough.

Activities of Life and Activities of Recreation

In the context of providing care or supervision for another, there are two categories of activity to define: activities of life and activities of recreation.

Activities of life essentially consist of Activities of Daily Living and Instrumental Activities of Daily Living. As discussed in previous chapters, Activities of Daily Living are personal care routines: bathing, dressing, eating, and toileting. Instrumental Activities of Daily Living are operational tasks necessary for preserving an independent lifestyle to maintain a household, involving everything from taking out the trash to scheduling appointments, and from financial record keeping to shopping. Instrumental Activities of Daily Living are routines that happen throughout life, regardless of age. These activities provide mental stimulation through decision making and problem solving, sometimes requiring careful thought as to how to accomplish tasks if adaptations to routines are necessary. Instrumental and Activities of Daily Living also promote independence by keeping a care recipient participatory in care schedules and decisions.

Activities of recreation fulfill physical, mental, emotional, and social needs. They are purposeful at any age or stage of life, even if they must be adapted to meet physical or cognitive functioning levels. Examples of recreation and leisure activities range from exercise programs to reading to card playing to arts and crafts. Recreational and leisure activities add quality to life, promoting a positive self-image that improves self-esteem. By participating, a care recipient uses physical and cognitive abilities to be productive and therefore achieves a sense of accomplishment. Especially in retirement years, recreational and leisure pursuits often replace workplace productivity; people look for ways to fill time with useful and meaningful activity. Activities that are group oriented encourage interaction and social connectedness.

The benefits of activities of life and activities of recreation can and do overlap. Grocery shopping (an activity of life) provides physical exercise if a care recipient is able to walk to the store and then through most of the aisles for additional exercise; even lifting foods and carrying grocery bags to the car can strengthen muscles. This may be the extent of exercise some care recipients receive. Light housekeeping (including dusting, vacuuming, and sweeping) is a mild form of exercise; raking leaves, sweeping the driveway, and cleaning windows will provide more aerobic benefits. These tasks may pose a health risk to some care recipients or at the least will be physically challenging; assistance should be offered or arranged for these care recipients. The care recipient who no longer manages bill paying or financial records will still feel productive and exercise cognitive skills (problem solving, mental stimulation) through recreational word and number games, such as crossword and math puzzles. Activities of life or recreation can maintain and improve mental and physical functioning.

A regular challenge for a care provider is to influence the home care recipient to become actively involved in activities around the home or in the community. Some care recipients do not feel they have time or energy to engage in recreational activities because they are consumed with recuperating from a medical condition or their regular routines have become more time consuming. Extra energy is directed toward maintaining personal care routines and the household, which are legitimate reasons. There may be other explanations for care recipients' lack of motivation. Use good judgment and only encourage activity involvement as the care recipient can tolerate. Combine activities of life with recreational activities, if only for exercise and sensory stimulation. Encourage the use of physical and cognitive skills; as much as possible, engage the care recipient in activities that stimulate or make use of the five senses.

Below are suggestions for getting a care recipient involved in activities around the house, outside of the house, or in the community.

Provide the care recipient with activity supplies and materials. If the care recipient enjoys crosswords, take a puzzle book or put it on the shopping list.

Take old garden magazines to care recipients whom you know enjoy plants and flowers, and pet magazines to animal lovers.

Cable television is acceptable though should not be used as a substitute for the care provider's responsibilities. In the 21st century, there are plenty of channels that offer educational and entertaining programs, covering topics of history, animals, cooking, old movies, travel, national geographic, and home decorating. Television should not replace what care providers can offer.

Use objects found in a care recipient's home as starts to conversation. Ask about people or places in photographs, paintings on walls, or flowers in the garden. Go through the care recipient's recipe collection or use a favorite cookbook to talk about foods and meals, and share your own.

Present new ideas without being forceful. The care recipient may not think to ask; providing thoughts may be just enough to stimulate involvement.

Initiate conversations and discussions about past and current areas of interest, and suggest activity ideas. Just talking with the care recipient may engage their interest.

Demonstrate how to do an activity. Many times, care recipients do not participate because they do not know how to perform the project. Offer simple directions or step-by-step instructions when appropriate. Be flexible, and allow the care recipient to apply his or her personal style.

Allow the care recipient plenty of time to complete an activity, especially if he or she is finding satisfaction with the process of doing rather than only finishing a project. In other situations, it just may take a care recipient longer than it once did to complete a given task or project.

Suggest taking the care recipient who likes to read to the library or book-store. If he or she declines or is unable, choose a book from the library you think the care recipient will enjoy. Music, movies, and books on tape can also be found at the library. This may motivate the care recipient to go along on the next trip.

If the care recipient will consider joining groups, such as an exercise or card club, suggest that he or she visit the facility or attend a session. The companion can accompany the care recipient, especially if the care recipient is shy or nervous.

A Companion's Role in Activity Planning

We already know that adding quality to life is the goal for the care provider and the purpose of activities is to make use of cognitive, physical, sensory, and social skills as much as possible. Planning or choosing activities depends on the care recipient's needs and abilities and the companion must understand how the purpose of the activity meets care recipient needs. It is helpful to know care recipient likes and dislikes, though trial and error works too.

Almost everything we do can be considered an activity, and almost all activities have purpose to life or recreation. One role of a care provider is to focus on the abilities and strengths of each care recipient, and turn tasks into activities. It is helpful and sometimes important to break down an activity into smaller tasks to understand how the activity is purposeful to the care recipient.

How do we choose effective, educational, and enjoyable activities?

Identify Needs

Recreational activities meet physical, cognitive, emotional, spiritual, and social needs. Observe, ask, and discuss with each care recipient which areas need attention. Is it advantageous for the care recipient to participate in group programs, or does he or she prefer solitary activities? Then prioritize needs as necessary and appropriate to make your activity creation more purposeful. Frequently, care recipients who are receiving companion or other home care will express what they feel is missing or lacking in their current situation and the desire to fulfill that need. Often care recipients want information, ideas, and guidance to get them started in recreational pursuits as a form of comfort.

Example: The identified needs for Client A are cognitive and social stimulation. Client A has difficulty with walking longer distances and needs to sit frequently.

Determine What the Care Recipient Is and Is Not Capable of Doing

Assess care recipients' physical and cognitive functioning, as physical limitations and cognitive impairments may dictate activities. When appropriate, ask the care recipient what feels too challenging. Also, consider how an activity might be adapted to accommodate compromised functioning levels. For example, if completing crossword puzzles is too challenging, suggest word finds; if walking longer distances is too strenuous though he or she still wants the exercise, make certain there are enough places to sit for periodic breaks.

> Example: It is determined that Client B is physically able to walk fair distances, though is moderately confused and forgetful.

Decide Where the Activity Will Take Place

Outings offer social stimulation and connection to the outside world, but this is not always practical or possible. There are plenty of activities of life and recreation that can and do happen in the home. Consider where the care recipient will be most comfortable and set up the appropriate situation. It is not very realistic to brush teeth in front of the television or chop vegetables in the bedroom! Word puzzles and reading can easily be done while sitting in a recliner, but if the care recipient will work on a picture puzzle, make space on the dining room table. If an outing is in order, decide on the best place to go based on past and current care recipient interests, as well as physical accessibility, costs, and crowds.

> Example: In earlier years, Client C volunteered at the art museum. To provide this client with opportunities for physical exercise, cognitive and social stimulation, and the ability to reminisce, taking a walk through the museum once a month is arranged.

Determine What Supplies or Materials Are Needed to Complete the Activity

To make activities successful, supplies may be needed. If the care recipient does not already own the necessary supplies, try to improvise; if there are no substitutes, talk with the care recipient about putting the items on a shopping list. Exercise routines do not require equipment; instead of weights, use canned vegetables or bottles of liquid, such as dish or laundry detergent. Preparing meals or snacks obviously requires necessary food items. Puzzle books, puzzles, cards, magazines, newspapers, and books are tools to stimulate cognitive skills. Craft projects, such as sewing or knitting, call for needles and yarn. If an outing is planned, maybe a trip to the bank is necessary to cover admission fees or other incidental costs.

> Example: A trip to the art museum requires a few items. Encourage Client C to wear comfortable clothes and walking shoes. Money for admission is needed, and enough for a snack or beverage may be wanted. Supplies indirectly needed for this activity could be an umbrella or coat, or even taking along snacks and beverages.

Evaluate the Activity

Is the in-home activity or outing a success? What made it work? Why didn't it work? What would have made it better? Ask the care recipient for positive and negative feedback to make future changes and adaptations with other care recipients. Remember, what works for one care recipient may not work for another, which is why it is important to go through the above steps one through four.

Example: The art museum was pleasing to Client C, who benefited from the walking exercise, social interactions, and seeing paintings that she always enjoyed—referring to them as "old friends." This was a perfect place to get out of the summer heat—just as perfect on a cold, snowy day too. There were plenty of benches throughout the museum to take the needed rest breaks, and sitting in the café drinking lemonade was an extra bonus on the trip. The outing was a success!

Client A, however, is not able to walk the distance of the art museum. In order to make it work for Client A, arrangements with the museum for a wheelchair will need to be made in addition to finding the elevator to access the second floor. Client A also lives on a tight budget; taking snacks and drinks from home is more sensible. This outing was also a success because individualized accommodations for Client A were considered.

Of course, there are plenty of activities that occur naturally and spontaneously, without much thought or planning. Such activities can be just as effective and enjoyable. Be flexible and question your definition of productivity: Perfect results are not always the answer. Especially when working with persons with Alzheimer's disease, where keeping the care recipient involved is more important than the outcome. It is more important that the care recipient has the opportunity to paint than what the completed picture looks like.

Be Prepared With Activities

A good practice is to prepare ahead with activity ideas before each visit. Keep a bag of supplies on hand with objects for discussion and use during visits. Fill the bag with the following, and every so often change the contents to add variety:

Reading material (books, magazines, newspapers) for the care recipient
Cards and other easily transportable games
Puzzles
Word puzzle and game books (i.e., crosswords, word finds)
Music cassettes, compact discs, or books on tape
Movie videos or DVDs
Paper, greeting cards, stationary
Pens, pencils, markers
Journal for writing stories together, or notes

Being prepared with activity ideas and supplies provides the companion with a course of direction for how to spend time with the care recipient (see Tip 8.1). An activity plan will make visits more successful. Furthermore, activities that are interesting to the care recipient *and* companion can prevent caregiver burnout by helping the companion not feel bored on the job, and providing the companion with a sense of purpose. Activities cultivate relationships; the action of doing things, and spending time together, provides opportunity toward a deeper understanding between the care recipient and companion.

Tip 8.1

Tips for Choosing Activities

Use familiar activities: Recognizable routines can promote participation with greater chances of the care recipient being able to accomplish the known activity

Incorporate exercise, with adaptations as needed

Emphasize multisensory experiences

Encourage activities that use social, physical, and cognitive skills: These activities stimulate intact skills

Use age, gender, and ability-appropriate activities: Monitor for too simple or too challenging activities, either of which can impact participation, accomplishment, and esteem

Give simple directions for completing a task or activity:

Initiate conversations involving reminiscing, which encourages the ability to recall past memories.

Use activities that are relevant to personal and professional experiences

Activity Ideas

The following section presents activity ideas, instructions, and the benefits of each activity. The activities are presented in seven categories common to relevance and recreational needs of care recipients:

Around the House
Exercise
Games
Music
Outdoors
Outings
Reminiscing

An overview of each category presents general information and purpose for initiating experiences, including what skills are used and how this benefits a care recipient. Activity ideas follow, which suggests the skills used in the activity, direction on how to complete the activity, and considerations for adapting the activity to meet individual care recipient needs.

Around the House

Purpose: To stimulate sensory, social, and physical skills, as well as cognitive skills through decision making and the ability to reminisce.

Description: Maintaining a household serves practical and purposeful reasons. Some household tasks, such as cleaning the kitchen and bathroom, are necessary for making the home fit for living. Cleanliness contributes to health and safety by reducing germs, which can lend to infection or illness, and minimizing the possibility of injury. Other tasks are done with pleasure or to fill a sense of pride; for example, gardening or indoor and outdoor decorating.

Without managing these everyday jobs and responsibilities, a care recipient may feel useless and unproductive. Encourage the home care recipient to participate in running the household as much as he or she is physically and cognitively able in order to improve his or her physical functioning, self-image, and well-being. Be aware that household responsibilities can be overwhelming to the care recipient. The care provider's role is a delicate balance of knowing when to persuade the care recipient to act independently and when to offer assistance, without creating dependency.

Household management uses problem-solving and decision-making skills, as well as fine and gross motor skills.

Case Study

April experimented with gourmet cooking as a hobby in her younger years and considered herself a "foodie": She was interested in new and exotic recipes, knew fun food facts, and kept up to date on new foods and products. A degenerative condition slowly diminished April's ability to ambulate with ease or comfort, and she stopped going to the grocery store. She created grocery lists, but was buying the same foods over and over; not being able to see new or familiar foods stifled her creativity in the kitchen and she lost interest in food and eating, resulting in weight loss.

In time, April used an electric wheelchair and was able to go shopping with a companion. The best part, April said, was feeling independent again and able to make informed choices. She looked forward to meal planning *and* going to the grocery store! Because she enjoyed eating, she ate better, healthier foods, and gained the weight she had lost.

Shopping

Purpose: To stimulate sensory, social, and physical skills, as well as cognitive skills through decision making and the ability to reminisce.

Description: There are a variety of places to shop: garden shops, groceries, bookstores, department stores, and home stores; pharmacies; even medical equipment supply stores. Encourage the care recipient to create a list of wants and needs before leaving home. Additionally, ask the care recipient where and what he or she prefers to buy and plan trips to these specific destinations. Be flexible and spontaneous! If you find another store while you're out and time permits, persuade the care recipient to visit a new store. Sometimes shopping is used for recreational reasons, just to get the care recipient out of the home and into a public place for sensory and social stimulation. Shopping also promotes the ability to reminisce. The care recipient may talk of how products and prices have changed over the years, the discovery of new products, or past shopping experiences.

Considerations: There are several ways to manage mobility issues. Many stores provide wheelchairs or electric scooters for use at no cost. A care recipient will operate the scooter independently, although instruction on how to control and maneuver it will be necessary. Chairs and benches can be found scattered throughout some stores; if there is no risk of a care recipient wandering away, allow him or her to sit while the companion collects the shopping items. Even this type of social stimulation can be advantageous to a care recipient.

To use shopping as a recreational activity for confused care recipients, walk them through the store on a treasure hunt. For instance, ask the care recipient to point out apples, oranges, and bananas in the produce area, or ask the care recipient to identify a couch, wreath, and lamp in a home goods department store. For the home care recipient who is unable or prefers not to leave home to shop and where computer access to the Internet is available, encourage online shopping. A companion may also provide care recipients with relevant web site addresses and information. Sufficient funds are needed to go shopping! Companions will not always know care recipients' financial positions, and purchasing decisions are usually not decided by a companion. If a care recipient is cognitively impaired or has impaired judgment, ask family members if there are spending rules or limits before the shopping trip.

Gardening

Purpose: Use of fine and gross motor skills, sensory and cognitive stimulation, and the ability to reminisce.

Description: Growing flowers, plants, and herbs does not only take place in an outdoor flower bed. All of these can be arranged in clay or plastic pots and placed in the yard or on sidewalks and porches. They do not have to be large or exotic, only appealing to the eye, and should be manageable for the care recipient and others who are tending to them. Plants and flowers should be used decoratively to lift spirits and add joy, not to become another troublesome household chore. An indoor houseplant can become an object for the care recipient to take care of, which can fill a sense of purpose and function. For care recipients unable to physically participate in outdoor gardening, suggest they water the garden or give them the necessary planting materials for container gardening: planter, dirt, and a flower start. If care recipients prefer to passively participate, set up a chair with a view for them to watch you work.

Considerations: If the care recipient has an outdoor garden and is unable to manage the physical labor of maintaining a garden, the companion can offer assistance with planting, watering, weeding, picking off fruits and vegetables (i.e., tomatoes), or cutting flowers for a fresh bouquet. If heavier work needs to be done, suggest hiring a lawn and garden service. Stimulate cognitive skills by asking care recipients to identify plant and flower types and ask care recipients to share memories related to flowers and gardening. Care recipients with cognitive impairments can benefit from such conversations as well as from the sensory (visual, tactile, and olfactory) perceptions.

Cooking or Baking

Purpose: Promotes self-sufficiency and independence; uses fine and gross motor skills; and involves sensory perception, cognitive skills, and social skills when working with another. Cooking or baking is an activity of life and recreation.

Description: Preparing an entire meal does not need to be difficult. Allow a care recipient to choose recipes; if a trip to the grocery store for ingredients is needed, consider taking him or her along for an outing. Encourage care recipients to do as much as they can, offering assistance only where needed. A companion may help by preparing the process by setting up ingredients, utensils, bowls for mixing, and pans for cooking. This could make meal preparation feasible for the care recipient to do independently. Care recipients can measure, mix and stir ingredients, or clean and chop ingredients. Other care recipients may need more assistance, where companions may need to open cans and bottles, cut fruits and vegetables, and oversee operations of the stove or oven. There may be situations where it is most helpful when the companion performs the entire meal preparation process, but a care recipient can passively participate by giving verbal directions or reading recipes aloud, or by making other conversation. Chapter 9 suggests how to plan and prepare meals, including recipes specific to limited diets.

Considerations: Care recipients with cognitive impairment or limited hand and arm mobility may need to be supervised when using sharp objects. If the companion is choosing the snack or meal, be sensitive to care recipients' likes, dislikes, diet restrictions, and food allergies. Properly store or refrigerate leftovers; to minimize food waste, be creative with the leftovers—meatloaf can turn into chili and tomatoes or corn can be added to chili or other stews, a chicken breast can be chopped into chicken salad, and partial fruits can be used on top of a lettuce salad.

Exercise

It is widely known that physical exercise significantly contributes to overall health and the prevention of illness or disease. Exercise maintains or builds bone density and muscle strength, keeps joints moving to maintain or increase mobility, and prevents weight gain, which can contribute to high blood pressure and other heart conditions. Certain types of exercises (walking, jogging) can improve cardiovascular (heart-related) health and the circulatory system. Research also shows that endorphins are released in the brain during exercise, contributing to mental and psychological health.

A care recipient who lacks proper exercise may feel depressed, sluggish, and tired, and a weight gain can negatively affect his or her self-image and esteem.

For the home care recipient, exercise can be walking from the bedroom to the kitchen, folding laundry, watering the outdoor garden, grocery shopping, lifting one to three pound hand weights, or other prescribed exercise routines. Exercise does not have to mean panting and sweating; it should be just enough to physically stimulate or elevate the care recipient's mood. The care provider should encourage as much activity as a care recipient will tolerate. Do not forget to allow him or her needed time to sit and rest; plus, encourage fluids (water is best) after activity.

Exercise provides physical stimulation by using gross and fine motor skills (i.e., hand-eye coordination). Social skills can be stimulated if the companion exercises with the care recipient. Cognitive and decision-making skills may be necessary if the exercise activity requires skillfulness, as with bowling or golf.

Outdoor Stimulation

Mary and her companion went to the neighborhood park to walk on the sidewalks along the river at least once a week, weather permitting. They played "kick the can" with empty soda cans or rocks while they walked to make use of hand-eye coordination, which also added innocent fun and laughs. In addition to the benefits of exercise, Mary interacted with children and adults, watched the river run, observed wildflowers, and took advantage of the opportunity to feed ducks. Benches were readily available, and taking rest breaks to sit and relax added to the experience. While sitting, they would reminisce, sing songs, and even play charades.

During inclement weather when they had to stay indoors, they exercised by walking laps around Mary's assisted living facility, sometimes kicking a beach ball (instead of a soda can) to exercise hand-eye coordination.

Walking

Purpose: To exercise gross motor skills and social and communication skills; to increase physical and mental stimulation.

Description: The physical act of walking needs little explanation, though there is room for creativity in why, where, and how to walk. Decide the reason for walking: Is it to get the care recipient in to a public place for socialization and stimulation, only for exercise, or a combination? Public areas for walking include parks, shopping malls, libraries, museums, and grocery and other stores. Encourage the care recipient to interact with children at the park—do not forget to seek permission from the parents! Or engage other adults in pleasant conversation. Add sensory and cognitive stimulation by pointing out your observations or asking the care recipient to identify what he or she sees. This is a wonderful opportunity to make walking a multisensory experience for a care recipient with Alzheimer's disease or dementia. For example, ask the care recipient to identify apples, green peppers, bread, and other products in a deli or bakery; or turn it into a game of I Spy: Provide the care recipient with the name of the object and ask them to find it. Walk indoors and out, repeating laps as needed to extend time exercising.

Considerations: Determine mobility issues and limitations and choose appropriate places to walk based on physical ability, familiarity, and past or current interests. Consider the art museum for care recipients who enjoy art, wander through a library or bookstore for those who enjoy reading, and try an outdoor community festival for those who are good walkers and like to be in social events. Indoor public places (i.e., shopping malls) are ideal on hot or rainy days. Using wheelchairs in place of walking still provides social and sensory stimulation; many public places loan or rent wheelchairs if the care recipient does not have personal equipment. If a fair amount of walking is anticipated, taking food and water may be appropriate.

Golf

Purpose: To exercise gross and fine motor skills, to increase physical and mental stimulation by focusing on hand-eye coordination and concentration, and to use social skills.

Description: Adapted forms of golf can be a physically low-impact sport. It is a fun activity to incorporate into an exercise routine, even if a care recipient did not play or enjoy golf earlier in life. Rather than playing an entire round (18 holes) of golf, consider an outing to the nearby putt-putt course; even then, play only as long as the care recipient can tolerate. Look for a public or private driving range as an outing, which allows people to stand in one place and hit a bucket of golf balls. If the care recipient enjoyed golf earlier in life but is unable to manage the walking or outdoor terrain of a putt-putt course or golf range, set up a similar one-hole game in the home by using a plate or glass (on its side) as the cup; for serious golf enthusiasts, suggest the purchase of a golf game found at a sporting good store—do take the care recipient along for an outing!

Considerations: Ask the care recipient if he or she belongs to a country club or golf club; if so, use those facilities. It is a good way to keep the care recipient in touch with familiar people and surroundings, helping him or her remain connected to a previous lifestyle. Mobility may be an issue, so be creative: Use a golf cart, place a chair at the tee on a driving range for rest periods, or practice putting on only one hole to minimize walking. Care recipients with canes, walkers, and wheelchairs may still be able to putt-putt or perform at the driving range with assistance.

Chair Exercises

Purpose: To stimulate fine and gross motor skills and hand-eye coordination.

Description: Exercising from a chair can strengthen arm, leg, and torso muscles while preventing a person from becoming off balance (when standing), which could result in a fall. There are numerous movements that can be used. To exercise arms and shoulders, try an imitation of rowing a boat, large and small arm circles, shoulder rotations, and extending arms up and out. To exercise the legs, do leg lifts (one leg at a time, then both together), knee lifts, kicking out, and marching in place. To promote flexibility, try neck, hip, wrist, and ankle rolls, and toe touching. Alternating movements between the upper and lower body, and between arms and legs, encourages endurance. When the arms or legs are exercised without a brief period of rest, they will tire quickly.

Considerations: Only exercise the care recipient as much as he or she is able to tolerate and be sure that exercise is approved by a physical therapist, nurse, or physician. Consider getting a chair-exercise, yoga, or tai chi video or DVD from the library, which could motivate a care recipient to exercise more if the routines are physically possible and appealing. Playing music during exercise makes for a pleasant experience. Write down and demonstrate specific movements so a care recipient can exercise during alone time. For care recipients who are able to lift light weights, 1–3 lb. hand weights can be purchased, or use household items as substitutes—a bottle of bleach or laundry soap can be just as effective for strengthening arm muscles.

Games

Playing games is an excellent way for a care recipient and companion to interact and build a relationship. They are a fun way to engage the care recipient and spend otherwise idle time. Older adults commonly use games for recreational and educational purposes. The board game Parcheesi requires little mental skill and would be used as recreation, while the games Scrabble and Chess require thinking, decision making, and planning. Card games can be mentally stimulating, and can be played individually or with others. Word games, such as crossword puzzles and word finds, are popular with older adults because they can be done when the care recipient is alone—most do not need more than one person, can be started and finished in short periods of time, and need few materials and supplies. There are numerous ways to use words as games. *The following activity ideas will focus on word games, including trivia, rather than cards or board games.*

Games offer mental stimulation through thinking, problem solving, and decision making. Social, communication, and verbal skills are exercised when games are played with more than one person. Many board games require fine motor skills by moving pieces and parts or rolling dice; other games may use gross motor skills.

Mind Mapping as a Recreational Tool

Meredith has lived alone for 8 years, since her husband died. She had never been active in the community and was satisfied spending time doing her own things. Her ideas for recreation and relaxation were watching soap operas and game shows, listening to oldies music, working picture puzzles, and doing word searches. She kept herself happily busy with these activities. Her family thought a companion would provide basic supervision and just enough socialization to not interfere with Meredith's personal routines.

Though polite and pleasant, she was not much of a conversationalist and the companion had a hard time getting Meredith to talk about herself. The companion decided to use mind mapping (an instrument often used in brainstorming sessions, see Figure 8.1 toward the end of this chapter) as a type of game to encourage Meredith to share memories. The map served as a visual tool showing Meredith's life experiences. While asking questions and writing the answers on paper, Meredith smiled as she remembered more memories and shared more stories.

The companion's game of getting to know Meredith worked, and she recognized the companion's effort and genuine interest in her life stories. With the help of the mind-mapping tool, Meredith and her companion formed a relationship that became the start of a faithful friendship.

Magazine Treasure Hunt

Purpose: To use cognitive and sensory skills and the ability to reminisce.

Description: Look through a magazine to create a list of objects found in the pictures. Give the list to the care recipient and ask them to find each item on the list. This activity can be done during the visit to promote social interaction or the list can be left with the care recipient to work on during alone time. Depending on the care recipient's functioning level and interest in this activity, create more than one list. For a challenging activity, create a list of words found throughout a magazine or a particular article.

Considerations: Use magazines with pictures and subjects that appeal to the care recipients' interests, such as history, gardening, or motorcycles. Home and garden magazines are well suited for persons with mild dementia or confusion because most objects in these magazines will be familiar and recognizable. Rather than creating lists and looking through magazines (especially if none are on hand at the time of the activity), adapt the treasure hunt to what is visible in the room. This is more appropriate for confused care recipients at home or in a facility. (For instance, ask "Where is a clock?" and have the care recipient identify a clock in the room.) Allow time for other conversations to occur; pictures may spark memories that the care recipient wants to share. This can also be a good opportunity for him or her to talk about current issues or concerns.

Word Games

Purpose: To exercise cognitive skills; includes the potential for the ability to reminisce and social stimulation.

Description: Word games come in a variety of forms: word searches, crossword puzzles, word scrambles, fill in the blanks, word associations, spelling, and trivia. Even number games such as Sudoku fall into the word game category. Work on word games together during visits or provide the care recipient with the games to do in alone time. Puzzle books of all varieties can be found at grocery stores, pharmacies, and book and dollar stores. Many newspapers have a game page with crossword puzzles and other word activities. The library will have trivia and game books, though writing in them is not acceptable; supply your own paper. A companion can easily and quickly create word-game activities at home with pen and paper:

Word scrambles: NPATL unscrambled is PLANT
Word associations or combinations: Birds and ____ (Bees)
Fill in the blanks: Red, White, and ___ (Blue)
Create new words from a phrase: use GARDEN FLOWERS to create dare, flow, safe, glow, etc.

Considerations: Word associations and fill in the blanks can be done without pen and paper, as can spelling bees and categories (Desserts: cookies, cake, pie, cupcake, etc.). Using categories: As an example, ask the higher functioning care recipient to create lists of presidents' names or television shows; with lower-functioning care recipients, keep categories simple with colors and animals. Vary the challenge of each word game based on care recipient's functioning level. Allow time for other conversations to occur; words may spark memories that the care recipient wants to share. This can also be a good opportunity for him or her to talk about current issues or concerns.

Puzzles and Board Games

Purpose: To stimulate cognitive skills and social skills, as well as fine motor skills and hand-eye coordination.

Description: Puzzles can be worked when a care recipient is home alone or with a companion as a social activity; most board games require at least two people. They come at varying skill levels and can be too easy or too difficult. Be aware of cognitive abilities: Do not insult a care recipient by suggesting a game that requires little skill if he or she is higher functioning; stop the activity if it is too challenging and the care recipient becomes frustrated. Follow the given directions of each game, though adapt as necessary to meet a care recipient's functioning needs. Large-piece puzzles are readily available at toy and drug stores and large grocery stores.

Considerations: Not every care recipient will want to play games or work puzzles, and there may not be any in the home. If the care recipient gives permission, offer to buy a game or puzzle on a shopping trip. For the care recipient who is not interested in a game or puzzle, encourage word games or reminiscing discussions to exercise cognitive and social skills.

Music

Melodies and songs have a way of stimulating memory to provoke thoughts, feelings, moods, and even physical reactions. Music can increase physical and mental stimulation or relaxation when used effectively. For instance, music helps to engage participants in exercise or physical movement activities; and calm, soothing music can be played for relaxation, to de-escalate tense situations, and to induce sleep or periods of rest. Music brings enjoyment to most people, which can enhance our connections with others as well as our own expression of thoughts and feelings. Music is especially effective when working with Alzheimer's or dementia care recipients. Used successfully, music will motivate and enhance the quality of life.

Music is multipurpose. Thoughts and memories are brought to mind, benefiting cognitive skills and the ability to reminisce. In group or public settings, music can energize interactions, making use of social skills. Many people dance or simply move to music, therefore using gross motor skills. If exercise routines are set to music, the use of fine motor skills can be applied. Additionally, religious or spiritual music can strengthen a connection to God or a higher power.

Seasonal Offerings Present Opportunity

A local shopping mall held holiday concerts in the atrium over the lunch hour every December. Betty's companion contacted the mall at the beginning of the month (or checked the event schedule online) to learn about the groups who would be performing and the times of each concert. Betty and her companion picked up a picnic lunch and took it to the mall to watch elementary school students or active older adults from senior centers perform dance routines to familiar songs and holiday carols. It seemed Betty was mentally transported to a happier place and time while simply enjoying the sights and sounds of the season at the concerts. Over the 2-hour lunch break, filled with visual and auditory pleasures, she was able to take her mind off of her physical and emotional challenges.

During summer months, Betty and her companion went to a downtown park every Thursday with a picnic lunch to listen and watch various musical groups perform. They spent 2 to 3 hours at the park eating, listening to music, watching children dance, and taking time to wander through the gardens to smell the flowers.

These indoor and outdoor music activities provided Betty with recreational opportunities for social interaction and physical stimulation, and occasions to recall fond memories.

Live Music

Purpose: To encourage the ability to reminisce; to promote calming techniques, relaxation, and enjoyment; to exercise social skills; and to increase movement or physical stimulation.

Description: Check with children's and senior citizen choirs and band groups for public performances. Schools frequently perform concerts that are open to the public. Churches and shopping malls often host holiday concerts, as do some public government buildings, such as the local courthouse or statehouse. Contact the offices to request a schedule or calendar of events.

Considerations: Do call the venue ahead of time to learn about accessibility for care recipients with mobility issues. If appropriate, take food or drink.

Music at Home

Purpose: To encourage the ability to reminisce and to promote calming techniques, relaxation, and enjoyment.

Description: The benefits of music are easily applied to the care recipient. During visits, play the care recipient's choice of music softly in the background as you work or talk. The companion can borrow compact discs or cassette tapes from the library, or take the care recipient to the library on an outing so he or she can choose. Music videos or DVDs—concerts or musicals—can also be borrowed from the library and used if the care recipient has the necessary equipment for viewing. Radio stations offer the same benefits, if one can be found that is pleasing to the care recipient. Some cable and public television channels show concerts or musicals; check the local listings.

Considerations: If financially feasible, encourage the care recipient to purchase a compact disc (CD) player; they come in an assortment of models and sizes. Small, portable players with headsets can be found at many drug stores; larger players can be purchased at electronic or discount stores. Think about the care recipient's ease with using the equipment—avoid too many bells and whistles. A basic player with the play, stop, forward, and backward buttons should be sufficient. Also, consider where the player is placed in the home: Make sure it is accessible to the care recipient for use when no one is in the home to assist.

Singing Songs

Purpose: Promotes the ability to reminisce and encourages social stimulation.

Description: During visits, learn what type of music and even specific songs a care recipient prefers. Talk about music and favorite songs from his or her past, and the memories associated with each song.

Considerations: Higher functioning home care recipients may find a sing-a-long too juvenile, so the care provider should be sensitive to care recipients' functional and recreational needs. For this type of care recipient, suggesting participation in church or community choirs could be more favorable.

Outdoors

The outdoors means something different to everyone. For some, being outside is sitting on the front or back porch listening to sounds of birds, neighbors, and traffic. Some home care clients do not even venture outside without supervision because of the potential for a fall. Many home care clients would welcome the chance to sit on the porch, take a trip through the yard, or a walk to the mailbox. For others, being outdoors means being more engaged with nature and being in nature, the world of living things, away from people and urban areas. Fresh air is good for the spirit, and oxygen can aid sleep.

Being outdoors is a multisensory experience. The senses of seeing, hearing, smelling, and touching are stimulated. The outdoors promotes cognitive and physical skills. Recognizing the various birds or trees requires cognitive ability and some degree of physical participation, usually walking, is required. Gross motor skills are needed to walk. Nature can evoke thoughts, memories, and feelings, making use of cognitive skills and the ability to reminisce. With a companion, the care recipient will use communication and social skills.

Enjoying the Outdoors From Inside

Mary had a fall that resulted in a broken hip. Fortunately, she was able to ambu-late with a walker after a period of therapy and rehabilitation. The fear of falling again restrained Mary; she limited her activities to those that did not present huge potential for another fall. The companion recognized these concerns and looked for interesting, low-impact activity ideas for Mary, who had spent plenty of younger years hiking. The companion wanted Mary to once again appreciate nature but knew of Mary's fears and concerns, so came up with an alternative.

Mary and her companion picked up a picnic lunch and headed to the nearby state park, which housed an extensive nature center. They toured the center, learning about local habitat, much of which Mary already knew and shared with her companion as they made their way through the center. One wall of the cen-ter was windows with a full view into a wooded area for watching birds. Above the windows were speakers, which allowed the singing birds and outdoor noises to be heard inside. Instead of sitting at the outdoor picnic area, they sat in the nature center to watch wildlife while eating, which relieved Mary's fear of walk-ing across the uneven ground. The multisensory experience of the outdoors was brought indoors, in a satisfying way, where Mary could enjoy it in comfort and safety.

Parks

Purpose: Promotes physical stimulation, sensory perception, and the ability to reminisce.

Description: An outing to a local park or preserve is the most obvious way to enjoy being outdoors. If the care recipient is physically unsteady or unable to walk on outdoor terrain, use a wheelchair, sit in the car at a park to enjoy the view, or drive through a natural, scenic area. It can be just as advantageous to place a chair by the window in the home for the care recipient to see the outside sights.

Considerations: Pack a picnic lunch and find an accessible sitting area to eat. Binoculars and bird or duck food will add to the outdoor experience. Be sure the care recipient is dressed comfortably and appropriately for weather conditions.

Conservatory (Greenhouse and Gardens)

Purpose: Supports physical exercise, and stimulates sensory and cognitive skills and the ability to reminisce.

Description: Conservatories often have outdoor floral gardens with art sculptures, greenhouses with exotic plants and flowers, indoor exhibits, and classes and demonstrations. In suitable weather, walk though the gardens and sit on benches to relax and observe the outdoors to stimulate visual, olfactory, auditory, and tactile perceptions. Touring the greenhouses and exhibits offers a multisensory experience, and is an excellent way to sense the outdoors dur-ing cold or rainy weather. For sensory stimulation, encourage a care recipient to smell and touch plants (as permitted by facility). Ask the care recipient to identify flower and plant types to stimulate cognitive skills. To rouse stories, ask care recipients about favorite flowers and gardening experiences.

Considerations: A picnic lunch or eating in an onsite café (if available) will contribute to a delightful outing. Consider taking a camera and compiling the pictures into a photo album so the care recipient will have a visual reminder of the outing. A trip to the conservatory usually entails a fair amount of walking; contact the facility in advance to learn if wheelchairs are available for public use. As always, be sure the care recipient is dressed appropriately with comfortable walking shoes. There may be an admission fee to enter the conservatory; call ahead to learn costs and hours of operation.

Garden Stores or Nurseries

Purpose: Uses gross motor skills, stimulates sensory and cognitive skills, and enhances the ability to reminisce.

Description: Walking through a garden center provides nearly the same benefits as visiting a conservatory. The multisensory experience stimulates the senses: sight, sound, smell, and touch. To stimulate cognitive skills, ask the care recipient to identify flowers and plants. Ask care recipients about favorite flowers and gardening experiences to encourage reminiscing.

Considerations: A garden store or nursery may be closer to home and easier to get around than a trip to the conservatory, and there is no admission fee. A nursery may be smaller than the conservatory, which would be beneficial for clients with mobility issues. Money will be needed if the care recipient wants to purchase flowers for the outdoor garden or household plants—tending to plants or flowers can be very therapeutic. Be sure the care recipient is wearing comfortable clothes and shoes.

Outings

Getting out of the house (or facility) can help a care recipient feel a sense of normalcy and connection to the outside world. Outings do not have to be extravagant; the purpose is to get the care recipient into public places to interact with people, and can be a form of exercise.

Cognitive, communication, and social skills are used during outings, which also stimulate the senses of seeing, hearing, smelling, tasting, and touching. Destinations can be reminders of past memories and may awaken particular thoughts and feelings. Gross motor skills are needed to walk, while fine motor skills may be necessary for some outing activities. Care providers should look for places and events that create multisensory experiences.

Food as Fun

Luckily, the town in which Violet lived was home to peanut butter, popcorn, and chocolate factories. Her companion rotated outings to each factory throughout the year.

They toured the plant floor of the peanut butter factory and talked with workers, who showed them the methods and equipment used to sort, clean, and roast nuts before they are processed into butters and spreads. At the chocolate factory, Violet and her companion observed the process for making chocolate and how it is shaped into bars and candies with molds. This was a long tour with a fair amount of walking, though seats were available for rest periods. At the popcorn factory, how the corn is popped in large poppers, then flavored and packaged, was demonstrated. Free samples were given at the end of each tour and Violet always wanted to stop in the gift shops so she could take chocolate, popcorn, and peanut butter home.

They continued to make trips to the factories even though Violet was becoming more confused due to Alzheimer's disease and was unable to comprehend the information provided in each tour. The companion knew that Violet still enjoyed interacting with others and walking indoors made exercise tolerable on hot and cold days.

(Note: look under "museums" in the yellow pages, check the calendar of events in the newspaper, and contact your local Convention and Visitor's Bureau to learn about attractions and places to visit in your area.)

Art Galleries and Gift Shops

Purpose: To exercise, participate in social interactions, and encourage sensory stimulation.

Description: Find an area of town that offers restaurants, retail shops, and art galleries within a short distance of one another. The advantage of having this variety of offerings close together is that physical, social, and sensory stimulation can occur in a short period. Start on one side of the street and walk a few blocks, depending on the care recipient's physical abilities. A nearby restaurant can provide a place to sit and relax when a rest is necessary. Indulge in a snack or plan ahead to eat lunch in the area.

Considerations: If the weather does not permit walking outside, consider an outing to an indoor shopping mall for the same benefits. Take a wheelchair in case the care recipient tires from walking. Money will be needed for food, drink, and shopping.

Quilt Stores

Purpose: Provides sensory stimulation, social interaction, and physical exercise.

Description: Visiting a quilt store is a good sensory experience, even for those who have never made a quilt. Materials and fabrics provide visual and tactile stimulation, and the patterns on completed quilts can be thought provoking. Some quilt stores hang finished quilts on the walls as artwork.

Considerations: Find other specific shops with subjects related to care recipient interests, such as athletic, book, or home stores. Consider walking aids (i.e., wheelchair) as needed, and money for care recipient purchases.

Museums (Art, History, or Other)

Purpose: Provides cognitive, physical, social, and sensory stimulation as well as the ability to reminisce.

Description: Museums make wonderful outings! They make information available to learn about a subject (cognitive stimulation) and usually exhibit objects for people to view and sometimes touch—visual and tactile stimulation. Some museums or exhibits encourage interaction with other participants that provide opportunities for social stimulation. Museums provide the place and space for indoor walking, which is ideal for days of inclement weather. Plan to spend a few hours at a museum; between viewing exhibits and taking rest periods from walking, time can pass quickly.

Considerations: Look under "museums" in the yellow pages or contact the local Convention and Visitor's Bureau (CVB) to learn about attractions and places to visit in your area. Ask the care recipient about particular subjects and areas of interest; take him or her to museums with relevant offerings. Encourage the care recipient to wear comfortable clothes and shoes. Call the museum in advance to learn cost of admission, hours of operation, wheelchair accessibility, and driving directions.

Reminiscing

To reminisce is to remember the past. It is the process of remembering experiences and memories. The goal of using reminiscence as an activity is to bring fond, not unpleasant, memories to mind. Reminiscing is a regular activity for people with Alzheimer's disease because it can help them recall familiar people, places, or events. Short-term memory is lost before long-term memory in Alzheimer's disease; therefore, long-term memories—events from the distant past—may be easier to access than short-term recollections. People who do not have memory impairment also find pleasure in talking about their past and bygone customs and traditions. The act of reminiscing serves to validate a person's life by rekindling thoughts and feelings of times when personal goals and achievements were being accomplished. It is through reminiscing that a companion will learn the care recipient's character—what, why, and how he or she participated in private and community life. Asking questions and participating in these conversations shows interest by the care provider, which will help build rapport with the care recipient.

The ability to reminisce stimulates cognitive skills through processing thoughts and memories. When sharing memories, a care recipient will exercise communication and social skills. Reminiscing can be sensory if the memories are about special sights, smells, sounds, tastes, or touches; or if the activity to evoke remembering makes use of the five senses. While reminiscing is important, it is also important to talk about current events with higher functioning care recipients to keep them living in the present and connecting with the world outside of the home.

Addressing Memories

After a short stay in the hospital, Trudy returned to her apartment in the assisted living facility. She had lower energy levels and was not quite ready to get back in the swing of the activity schedule she maintained prior to the hospitalization.

Trudy did not leave her room except for meals, so her family decided to temporarily hire a companion to keep her company until she got back on her feet.

During a visit, the companion noticed Trudy's address book sitting next to the telephone. The companion thought reading the names aloud from the address book would start conversation and create opportunities for Trudy to share stories. It also served as a way for the companion to get to know Trudy. The companion started at names beginning with *A* and went through to *Z*, which took over an hour. Trudy was thrilled to share memories and stories of her family and friends! The familiar names reminded Trudy of her high school and college days, and the companion learned what Trudy did and thought during different periods of her life. They talked about her cousins and relatives of James, her deceased husband. Many names in the address book were of friends who Trudy and James saw every year when they vacationed at their beach house. Trudy joyfully recalled memories of the times she and James had shared with their friends on summer vacation. The reminiscing activity was successful: Trudy told the companion about her career, her happy life with her husband, and their children and travels.

Sending Cards for Birthdays, Celebrations, and Holidays

Purpose: Promotes the ability to reminisce, provides social stimulation, and uses fine motor skills (if care recipient is actually writing).

Description: Writing and sending notes, letters, and greeting cards is an excellent approach for prompting a care recipient to recall past memories of people, events, and occasions. Ask how the person who will be receiving the card is important to the client. Are there interesting stories of the card recipient? Are there specific memories of holidays, birthdays, or other celebrations with the card recipient? Sending cards promotes social interaction and the means for staying in touch with people who have been important to the care recipient. People who receive cards feel cared about and the people who send cards feel they are contributing to the happiness of others.

Cards or notes may be purchased, or created at home. Creating cards can but does not have to be an extensive craft project, keep it simple. Spending time with a care recipient making a card, assisting in composing a message, or talking about a letter the care recipient has already written opens up opportunities for reminiscing discussions.

Considerations: Plan a shopping trip so that the care recipient can choose greeting cards or supplies to make his or her own. Encourage the care recipient to purchase several or a box of mixed greeting cards to have on hand. An available supply of cards may motivate the care recipient to initiate his or her own activity to send cards more often. If the care recipient is physically unable to write a legible letter, offer to write it using his or her own words and sentiments.

Reminiscence Discussion Topics

Purpose: Provides social stimulation and encourages the ability to reminisce and recall. (Additionally, it is a chance for the companion to learn about the care recipient.)

Description: Reminiscing occurs on two levels: It can be recollections of the care recipient's personal stories, or of societal or worldly events that influenced a designated time period. (For example, World War II–era adults may recall food rationing and large numbers of women entering the workforce in addition to their personal experiences of serving in the War.) It can take place nearly anywhere and last 5 minutes or 5 hours, depending on how much information a care recipient wants to share. If it seems a care recipient does not want to share stories, allow him or her that privacy; change the subject or find another activity. Be casual and conversant: The care recipient does not need to know that a reminiscing activity is about to take place. Let it occur naturally.

To get ideas for discussion topics, look around the room or environment and ask questions about what you see. Is there an old photograph of people that could start a conversation about family members or past events? Does the house have antiques that may have unique stories? Is the care recipient wearing jewelry that could have been passed down through family generations? Newspapers, books, and magazines may also provide ideas for conversation starts. The following suggestions can also be used:

> Favorites: recipes, restaurants, bakeries, foods, sports teams, songs, movies, characters
> Firsts: day of school, date, dance, job, child, house, car
> Hobbies and use of recreational or leisure time
> Wedding day or other significant celebration
> Heroes and idols
> Accomplishments
> Vacations
> School
> Pets/Animals
> Work experiences
> Presidents and First Wives
> Political events
> Childhood house or neighborhood
> Current events, drawing comparisons to past events

Another interesting way to combine reminiscent and relevant discussions is to find a current product or process and ask the care recipient how it has changed over the years. The old story of what life was like before sliced bread is widely used as a metaphor to demonstrate the change of times. Computers and other technologies have changed the way we do things, and this change is occurring at a rapid pace. For the care recipient who creates shopping lists for others to use for running errands, suggest that he or she visit Web sites on the Internet to learn about product prices, availability, and variety. Practically, this is a form of shopping from home! Not only can this be an effective way to choose needed items, but it also evokes conversations of how things used to be and how they are now. This exchange of information can be particularly helpful to home care recipients who use previously established patterns that have become outdated in our fast-changing world.

Considerations: Pictures and photos from magazines, calendars, and personal collections can be used during reminiscing activities. Using pictures of familiar objects can be helpful when working with dementia and Alzheimer's care recipients.

Mind Mapping

Purpose: Promotes the ability to reminisce, provides social stimulation, and utilizes fine motor skills (if care recipient does the actual writing).

Description: This is an interactive, conversational tool that puts a care recipient's memories into words and onto paper. These maps provide visual cues for reminiscing; seeing familiar words written may encourage the care recipient to participate actively in sharing memories. A mind map starts with a simple word or phrase written in the middle of a piece of paper; thoughts prompted by that concept are written like spokes off of the initial word. Details provide more topics of conversation and when written create a spider web diagram. They can be brief or detailed, depending on how many memories and how much information a care recipient wants to share. It is not necessary to write entire stories or experiences; short phrases and words will suffice. A sample mind map is presented in Figure 8.1. The questions in this sample are suggestions and can be substituted.

Considerations: This tool can be adapted by using general instead of personal information. The initial word or concept could be of a category and associations or whatever comes to mind can be added to create the weblike appearance.

Summary

Thoughtful and purposeful activities add quality to life by providing mental, social, and physical stimulation. (A list of activities can be found in Tip 8.2.) Effective activities are multisensory; care providers should try to incorporate as many of the five senses (seeing, hearing, smelling, tasting, and touching) as

Tip 8.2

Alternative Activities

The following activity ideas can be used to stimulate moderately to severely impaired persons, and are easily adapted to meet a care recipient's functioning abilities. A care recipient may need help setting up the activity, though be able to perform the task independently. For example, a care recipient may not be able to retrieve items from the dryer but can fold them without further assistance. Other care recipients may need demonstrations or step-by-step instructions. Be attentive when supervision is necessary.

Household
Vacuum
Sweep
Dust
Wash dishes
Sort and fold clothes and towels
Water houseplants
Fill bird feeder
Retrieve mail

Cooking
Bake pies, cakes, or cookies
Decorate cakes or cookies
Prepare sandwiches or salads
Cut fruit or vegetables
Create ice cream sundaes

Exercise
Walk
Ball or balloon toss
Dance
Chair arm and leg stretches

Reading
Newspapers
Magazines
Novels
Short stories
Poems
Fairy tales

Games
Board games
Playing cards
Sorting cards by suits or numbers
Fill in the blanks
Word associations
Spelling bee
Categories

Other
Music
Cut out pictures and make a collage or scrapbook
Sort and count objects
Interact with children
Give a hand massage
Identify objects in the room

Example of a mind map. When mind mapping with a client, there is no need to write the question: It is the answer that spurs conversation. The written answers become the visual aid for stimulating social interaction and reminiscence

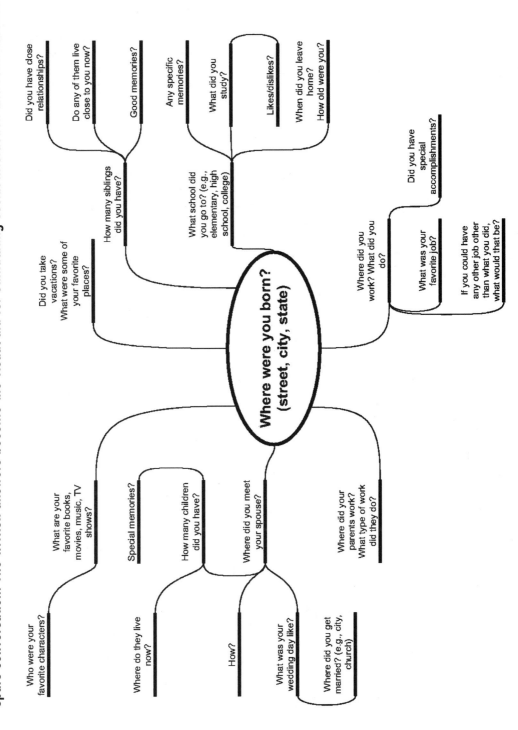

possible into one activity. Care recipients will benefit from both active and passive participation; providers should encourage care recipients' full participation while being sensitive to abilities and limitations.

Activities of life are Activities of Daily Living and Instrumental Activities of Daily Living. These are activities that maintain and support a care recipient's daily personal and household routines. Activities of recreation fulfill physical, mental, emotional, and social needs. They are important at any age or stage of life, even when they are adapted to meet physical or cognitive functioning levels. Care providers should motivate care recipients to participate to the best of their ability in purposeful activities of choice that encourage self-sufficiency, independence, and confidence.

Questions

What is the essential ingredient for creating successful recreational opportunities?
Give three examples of activities that support active or passive participation.
How can listening to music become an active participation activity?
What creates a multisensory experience?
Why are multisensory activities necessary?
What are seven categories of recreational opportunity?
Why is it important to understand the purpose and benefit of an activity?

Summary Tips

Ask questions and spend time getting to know care recipients' current and past interests.
Keep activity in range of care recipient abilities and limitations.
Activities with purpose will be more successful than activities that only serve to fill empty time.

Helpful Web Sites

Activities for elderly: http://www.righthealth.com
Activity ideas for activity professionals: Eldersong at http://www.elder song.com
Activity resources: ActivityResources.org at http://www.homestead.com/ac tivityresources
Educational activities for the elderly: Recreative Resources at http://www. recreativeresources.com

Suggested Reading

Cohen, Gene. (2001). *The creative age: Awakening human potential in the second half of life.* New York: HarperCollins Publishers. History, science, and true-life stories about human vitality and creative powers that come with age and experience.
Fisher, Pauline Postiloff, & Goldman, Connie. (1995). *More than movement for fit to frail older adults.* Baltimore, MD: Health Professions Press. Creative activities for body, mind, and spirit.

Keller, M. Jean. (1999). *Caregiving—leisure and aging.* Philadelphia: Haworth Press. Recreation and leisure needs of the older caregiver of an older adult.

Nekola, Pat. (2003). *Elder activities for people who care.* Waukesha, WI: Applewood Ink Publishing House. Activity planning and tips with the aging population.

Sheridan, Carmel. (1989). *Failure-free activities for the Alzheimer's patient.* San Francisco, CA: Elderbooks. Activity ideas for professionals and caregivers.

Walker, Susan. (1994). *Keeping active.* Atascadero, CA: Impact Publishers. A caregiver's guide to doing activities with the elderly.

Planning and Preparing Meals

9

In This Chapter, You Will Learn

1. Nutritional needs of the aging body

2. What special diets are and when they are appropriate

3. Signs of poor nutrition in an older adult

4. How to make meal planning an Instrumental Activity of Daily Living

5. How to create a pleasant dining experience

Why This Matters

Breakfast, lunch, or dinner may be the most momentous event in a day for an aging adult in the home or in a facility. The act of choosing foods and eating is one of the few sources of pleasure for many older adults. For some, deciding what, when, where, and how to eat is the only opportunity to make independent decisions. Eating is a personally satisfying experience when an individual creates a meal with foods of choice and a social activity when sharing a meal with others. Shopping, planning, and preparing meals is a recreational activity if the care recipient is able. Meal planning and preparation is an ideal occasion to show a care recipient respect by providing opportunities with choices and allowing autonomy. Eating is also necessary for good nutrition; obviously, food provides essential vitamins, minerals, and nutrients. Home care providers can educate care recipients about healthy foods and diet limitations to make informed decisions possible. Care providers should persuade care recipients to comply with special diets while balancing the care recipients' need to make independent decisions. Really, is it not acceptable for a mature adult to eat dessert first?

Nutrition, Eating, and the Aging Body

The need for a healthy diet does not decrease with age. In fact, inadequate nutrition and dehydration in older age are common problems that result in serious health consequences. The basal metabolic rate (BMR), which measures the minimal calories needed when a body is at rest, slows with age and the body does not need to consume as many calories for needed energy. Less activity is common in older age and the physical wants or needs for food may decrease.

There are several factors that contribute to unhealthy diets and poor nutrition. It may be difficult to physiologically digest foods properly, therefore causing stomach or intestinal problems. Foods may not agree with the body as they once did. To avoid discomfort, a person may keep away from those food choices. Signs that a person has a poor diet or lacks nutrition can be weight loss, low energy, tiredness, frequent infections, and wounds that heal slowly. Poor lifelong eating habits reveal results through various physical and physiological conditions, such as dental problems and diabetes.

Some elders who live independently may have trouble accessing healthy foods, whether because they are not able to get to the grocery or cannot afford to hire someone to do the shopping. Fresh produce and other foods considered healthy tend to be more expensive, which could limit these better purchases.

Taste buds change as we age or possibly as a result of illness and medications. Many people with cancer and other illnesses find they do not enjoy favorite foods as they once did and may be limited to certain foods that agree with taste and the body's reaction. People with Alzheimer's or dementia may forget what foods they like or dislike. One care recipient with late-stage Alzheimer's forgot she did not like broccoli or bananas; after moving into an Alzheimer's care unit, she ate them regularly. For another care recipient, adding artificial or natural sugar to foods was the only method to persuade her into eating nutritious foods.

Care providers should observe home care recipients' mealtime habits. For example, it is good practice to monitor weight, preferred portion sizes, how much food is not eaten per serving, and changes in amounts or types of food eaten. Observations and changes in habits should be reported to other appropriate care providers. Be aware of foods that can increase the risk for choking, such as hot dogs, and notice which foods cause individual care recipients problems with chewing, swallowing, or other types of reactions. A care provider should be cautious when suggesting diet provisions that may improve symptoms of a particular condition and should encourage the care recipient to discuss diet-related matters with a nurse, physician, or dietician.

Special Diets

There are several types of diets designed for special needs. Special diets can be prescribed to anyone, living anywhere. Care recipients who live independently in their own homes and residents of nursing homes may be placed on diet restrictions. It is typical for a speech therapist to evaluate the functional eating abilities of a person and recommend an appropriate diet while dieticians, nurses, and physicians make recommendations that meet dietary needs.

Various diets are available to meet the functional ability to eat. More common to nursing home residents are the mechanical-soft, puree, and thickened-liquid diets. The *mechanical-soft* diet is regular foods with a changed consistency for easier eating and chewing and does not have to mean less sugar, salt, fiber, or other nutrients. The diet includes well-ground meats and vegetables, mashed potatoes, pudding, and soft canned fruits or vegetables. Care recipients who have difficulty swallowing or chewing because of weakness as the result of a stroke, advanced Alzheimer's, or other neck and throat conditions do better on this soft-food diet. Mechanical-soft diets are also appropriate for people with digestion or dental problems, including dentures or no teeth at all. A *pureed* diet is similar to the mechanical-soft in that it is regular foods, with or without limitations on sugar or salt, but crushed in the blender to a smooth consistency that does not require chewing. *Thickened liquids* are liquids that have been thickened with a formulated powder provided by a nurse or dietician. It is not an additive to be created with home ingredients. Care recipients with swallowing disorders tend to aspirate, meaning the food or drink may enter the lungs causing aspiration pneumonia. Thickened liquids reduce this risk.

A unique type of special diet is the finger-food diet, usually applied to persons in mid- to late-stage Alzheimer's disease or with dementia. Finger foods are foods that are eaten easily with the hands: sandwiches, chicken fingers, cheese and crackers, cut vegetables, and cookies. Many mid- to late-stage patients with Alzheimer's are easily distracted and are unable to remain sitting for a meal. This diet offers nutrition on the go: The care recipient can eat while walking or pacing. It is also used for social reasons. When a care recipient is unable to properly and politely use utensils (fork, knife, or spoon) due to confusion, he or she will present inappropriately and therefore seem undignified when eating. In later stages of Alzheimer's disease, many people do not have the concept of utensils and will use their fingers to eat spaghetti, meatloaf, and peas. However, finger-food diets do not work with every person with Alzheimer's disease or dementia. A care recipient in mid-stages of Alzheimer's disease who had been raised with utmost manners would only use utensils, not fingers, to eat. In her confused state, she tried eating sandwiches and cookies with a fork or spoon. When she moved into an Alzheimer's unit, the staff was informed that she was not choosy about foods but that she must have foods she could eat with a fork or spoon.

Other special diets relate to health and dietary needs. The *diabetic diet* is a common special diet. This diet monitors the amounts of sugars and carbohydrates per serving; just as imperative is the portion of each serving. A low-sugar and low-carbohydrate diet may also be used as a weight-loss diet, whether or not the care recipient is diabetic. A *low-sodium* diet monitors salt intake. Red meats, prepared foods, frozen foods, and canned foods are notorious for high levels of sodium. People with a history or current condition of high blood pressure, strokes (CVAs), or heart conditions are likely candidates for this diet. *Low-fat* diets are also prescribed for people with heart conditions or history of strokes to reduce cholesterol and calorie intake. A *liquid diet* is just that: liquids such as broth, soup, tea, juice, and water. Jell-O is often allowed. Caffeinated products, such as colas and coffee, are not considered appropriate liquids for this diet and may be restricted. Care recipients on dialysis may have to follow a restricted diet that is unique to this procedure. If a care recipient is receiving this treatment, a care provider should be aware of these diet restrictions. Special diets are also used for cultural and social reasons, not necessarily for medical or therapeutic reasons. The vegetarian diet is gaining popularity in America as the significance of food as it relates to health is becoming more evident. There are at least two types of vegetarians and vegetarian diets. A vegetarian does not eat meat but will eat eggs and dairy products and a vegan does not consume any type of animal product. The Jewish Kosher diet is strictly followed in Orthodox Judaism. A noteworthy law of the Kosher diet is to not combine or serve meat and dairy products at the same meal, nor should meat and dairy be eaten within 6 hours of each other. If the client is Jewish and practices the Kosher diet it is extremely important to learn the food laws. As with other special diets, a care provider should understand and oblige client preferences.

A care provider should be aware of care recipients' diet restrictions in order to monitor diet compliance and issues. It is also important information if a care provider is doing the grocery shopping and meal preparation. Home care providers should realize that not all care recipients follow doctors' orders. Many care recipients are noncompliant and will not agree to obey the limitations of a special diet. This is a challenging situation for a care provider, especially if the care recipient is independent with decision making. The best approach to take with a care recipient who is not cooperating with diet restrictions is to educate him or her as to why the special diet has been prescribed. The care provider can recommend foods and beverages that are acceptable to the diet and delicately explain potential causes of harm if the diet is not followed. The care recipient will be able to make informed decisions with complete and accurate information; whether or not the diet is followed is another matter. An 82-year-old care recipient, who lived in her own apartment and managed her own affairs, attended a day care center 5 days a week. She had frequent hospitalizations resulting from her chronic diabetic conditions, though she continued to eat nearly a pound of candy a day. The social worker and nurse collaborated to educate the care recipient about proper food choices. The care recipient said she was well aware of her diet restrictions but was choosing to eat what she *wanted* rather than what was necessary for better health. The care recipient had the needed information to make better decisions for her health but made her own choice.

Grocery shopping for a care recipient on a restricted diet can present awkward situations for the care provider, particularly when the care recipient requests food items that are not permitted on the special diet. If a diabetic care recipient asks the care provider to pick up cookies, ice cream, and bread products, what should the care provider do? How does a care provider manage situations when care recipients, who are independent with decision making, consistently request groceries that are high in sodium when they have already had a stroke or suffer from high blood pressure? This type of situation is a common dilemma: Is it better for the care recipient to eat prepared meals with meats and vegetables—even if they are high in sodium—than to eat nothing at all? It is difficult to tell the independent care recipient what he or she can and cannot and should and should not buy, though the care provider should suggest foods that are suitable to the diet. The care recipient should be educated about nutritious foods and dietary guidelines. This is called educated or informed decision making—when the care recipient has needed information to make good decisions. Whether the care recipient takes the advice or not is uncontrollable, yet the information is available for him or her to decide what is of best interest. The care provider's role is to make the information available and assist with menu planning and shopping. (See "Cooking or Baking" under Activity Ideas in chapter 8.) If a care recipient is on a special diet or has diet restrictions because of medical treatments or conditions, consult with the doctor, nurse, or dietitian for individual needs.

Dietary Guidelines

The U.S. Department of Agriculture (USDA, 2007) has created American dietary guidelines to promote healthy eating and a well-balanced diet, which are updated every 5 years. These guidelines present a tool for planning nutritious meals and snacks and recommend minimum serving amounts from the food groups for daily intake of necessary nutrients, vitamins, and minerals. Consuming the suggested daily serving amounts is more important than the number of meals eaten every day. The following USDA recommendations are based on a 2,000-calories-a-day diet.

> Fruits: 2 cups, four servings
> Vegetables: 2½ cups a day
>
>> dark green: 3 cups a week
>> orange: 2 cups a week
>> legumes (dry beans and peas): 3 cups a week
>> starchy vegetables: 3 cups a week
>> other vegetables: 6 cups a week
>
> Whole grains (wheat, grain, and rye breads and crackers, unsweetened cereals, and brown rice): 3 ounces a day
> Milk and milk products: 3 cups a day
>> Meats and beans: 5.5 ounces a day

Vitamins and Minerals

The body does not absorb certain nutrients as readily in older years, which may require an increase in the amounts of needed vitamins and minerals, such as B-12 and calcium. Researchers have found that vitamin D contributes to the absorption of calcium and that they should be taken together. The body produces vitamin D with even minimal exposure to the sun; even 10 minutes is beneficial for the body to produce vitamin D. Foods rich in calcium are milk, cheese, yogurt, broccoli, leafy greens, canned salmon, sardines, and soybean products. Vitamin B-12 specifically helps form red blood cells. It is necessary for healthy blood and plays a role in preventing some cancers and improves functioning of the nervous system. A deficiency in B-12 can contribute to memory loss, confusion, depression, and coordination, all common symptoms in the aging experience. Food sources high in B-12 are lamb, beef, and pork livers and kidneys. Other good sources of B-12 are beef, egg yolks, milk, cheese, salmon, sardines, crab, and oysters. Vitamin A improves the immune system, reduces infections, and promotes healthy skin. It is found in animal sources including fish oil (from cod, halibut, and salmon), beef and chicken liver, and eggs. Another vitamin, C, also boosts the immune system to fight diseases, infections, cardiovascular disease, and some cancers. It can also help manage physical or mental stress. Foods containing high amounts of vitamin C are: broccoli, brussels sprouts, collard greens, kale, spinach, sweet peppers, cabbage, cauliflower, citrus pulp, and strawberries. Vitamin E is well-known as an antioxidant and is felt by many to be a miracle supplement. Research suggests the vitamin prevents some age-related diseases and conditions, such as cardiovascular disease and some cancers. Vitamin E may help wounds heal and it is believed to eliminate scarring when used as a gel or lotion. Vitamin E may also have a role in improving the immune and nervous systems, and for managing symptoms of diabetes. Many people take this vitamin as a supplement though high amounts are found in vegetable oils, including cottonseed, corn, safflower, soybean, and wheat germ. Smaller amounts of vitamin E can be found in legumes, nuts, whole grains, and dark leafy vegetables.

Fiber
Fiber aids in healthy digestion by lowering cholesterol, stabilizing blood sugars, and improving bowels and the intestinal system. Fiber can help prevent constipation and hemorrhoids. Fluids flush fiber through the body; it is imperative to drink plenty of water when eating fiber-rich foods. Many people take fiber supplements though it is found in whole grain cereals, rice, bran, fresh fruits, dried prunes, nuts, beans, peas, and fresh raw vegetables.

Protein
The body is energized by protein. It is essential for the body's cellular and tissue growth and development, which will aid the healing of wounds. Foods rich in protein are beef, fish, poultry, pork, cheese, eggs, milk, and yogurt; beans and nuts combined with rice also provides a rich source of protein.

Calcium
Many older adults lack adequate calcium and may have difficulty absorbing calcium. Calcium helps muscles and blood vessels contract and expand, and secretes hormones and enzymes that send messages through the nervous sys-

Tip 9.1

Monitoring Meals and Nutrition

Is the home care recipient at risk for inadequate or poor nutrition? Assess the situation every month, more often if there are noticeable changes in weight and eating habits. Report these changes to other care providers, family members, and the nurse or doctor. If the care recipient is able to understand your observations and concerns, discuss the matter directly with him or her.

Ask the following questions:

Has there been a loss of appetite without significant cause?
If so, for how long: days, weeks, or months?
How have eating habits changed?
Has the client changed the types or amounts of food eaten?
Has there been a weight loss?
Does the client have difficulty chewing or swallowing?
Is the client on a special or restricted diet?
Does the client have known food allergies?
How many meals a day does the client eat?
Does the client eat nutritious, healthful foods?
Does the client intake adequate water and fluids?
Where does the client eat?
Is the eating experience pleasing to the client?
Does the client eat alone?
Would the client benefit by having companionship during mealtime?
Are there noticeable times of the day that the client is or is not hungry?

tem. Foods rich in calcium are cheeses, milk (whole, skim, or 1%), orange juice, yogurt, ice cream, and leafy green vegetables (see also Tip 9.1).

Involving the Client in Meal Planning and Preparation

Food and eating is one of the last joys for some aging people. Mealtimes should be fun and enjoyable. Engage the care recipient in meal planning and preparation as an activity. The following ideas are adaptable to a care recipient's functional abilities:

Looking through grocery ads to create grocery list
Cutting coupons

Grocery shopping with caregiver
Finding favorite recipes
Measuring ingredients
Stirring/mixing ingredients together
Washing and chopping fruits, vegetables, meats, or other items
Spreading butter or jelly on bread
Reheating/cooking foods in microwave
Washing and drying dishes
Folding dishcloths and towels
Sorting silverware
Wiping the table and counters

For the care recipient who is unable to physically or cognitively prepare foods, he or she can participate by conversing with the person who is preparing foods and giving verbal directions and reading aloud recipes, or even the newspaper.

Preparing Meals

Cleanliness is the first rule of thumb when preparing meals: Hands should be washed, and all utensils, counters, and eating areas should be thoroughly cleaned before and after use. Fresh fruits and vegetables should be washed. Foods should be prepared according to package directions with necessary adaptations to meet specific diet restrictions. For example, if the package or recipe calls for one tablespoon of salt, consider using less or none at all. Amounts and serving proportions should be accurately measured particularly if the care recipient is on a special diet. Quickly cover and store foods that require refrigeration; periodically, clean out the refrigerator and discard older and spoiled foods.

Serving Meals

The second rule of thumb at mealtime: Create a pleasant dining experience. Eating is the activity, so allow the care recipients plenty of time to enjoy the meal. An unpleasant dining experience can lead to the care recipient eating less or nothing at all if they do not enjoy the food or ambiance, which can result in less intake and poor nutrition. The dining area should be kept clean and uncluttered; if practical, place fresh-cut flowers on the table. Place items such as salt, pepper, sugar, ketchup, and other condiments on the table during the meal for a care recipient who has difficulty with mobility (see also Tip 9.2). A care recipient may prefer to watch television or play music during meals. A care provider may not eat with the five o'clock newscast, but maybe the care recipient has eaten every dinner in front of the television for 20 years. Be considerate of care recipients' habits and routines. Many people find dining with others more pleasurable while others prefer to eat alone. The care provider should ask the care recipient's preferences and schedule visits during meals to offer companionship as appropriate.

Tip 9.2

Assistance During Meals

There may be occasions when a care provider will need to assist with feeding a care recipient who is in bed or bed bound. To avoid accidents and create a safe eating experience under these circumstances, consider the following:

Persuade the care recipient to sit upright, as close to a 90-degree angle as tolerated
Prop the head with pillows
Have ample table space next to the bed or an over-the-bed table
Allow plenty of time to eat; do not rush feeding
Cut food into small, bite-size pieces
Fill cups halfway or use straws
Place a towel over the chest to catch food or drink spills
Use a damp towel or cloth as a napkin
Keep extra towels or napkins nearby in case of spills
Use eating aids as appropriate
Encourage client to feed self as able

Shopping for the Client

Care providers often grocery shop when a care recipient is no longer able. Before every grocery shopping trip with care recipients, prepare and review the list and ask for specifics. For example, if bread is on the list, ask what brand, how many loaves, and what type: for example, wheat, white, rye, or seven grain. When potato chips are on the list, ask what brand (Lays, Conn's, Pringles, other), what size (small, medium, or large), what flavor (BBQ, Salt and Vinegar, Ranch, other) and how many bags. The idea of purchasing potato chips just became more complicated! Other considerations: Look for sell-by dates or dates of expiration and consider costs. If a care recipient is not particular about brands, ask if a generic or store-brand product is acceptable. Also, consider salt substitute, low-fat, and low-sugar alternatives, though ask the care recipient before purchasing other choices. Quality care providers consider and offer options so a care recipient has choices. This is a small step toward allowing the care recipient to maintain control and participate in decision making.

Following is a sample grocery list with items common to most lists. Would you know what and how to buy the following groceries?

Lettuce
Tomato
Potato

Bread
Soft drinks
Milk
Orange juice
Coffee

There are three significant reasons for clarifying details of the grocery list. First, if the care recipient is on any type of special diet, the purchased product should be permitted on that diet. If the care recipient is diabetic, diet soda pop is more acceptable; generally, full-sugar sodas are not part of a diabetic diet. A care recipient on a low-salt diet has similar concerns though must monitor salt intake. It is also helpful to be aware of known food allergies. The second reason is to understand care recipient likes, dislikes, and preferences so a care provider can offer quality service. The third purpose for reviewing the grocery list is to keep the care recipient involved in daily decisions and routines. Meal planning is an Instrumental Activity of Daily Living (IADL), a form of independence and self-determination.

A basic grocery list is provided below with specific questions to consider before setting out to the store.

Lettuce: What type? (iceberg, spinach, romaine, etc.) Does the client want it in a head or in a bag already cut up and ready to eat? Some clients may not be able to physically manage cutting lettuce. The modern convenience of bagged lettuces may encourage a care recipient to eat more salads.

Tomato: What kind? (cherry, beefsteak/sandwich, roma, etc.) How many? How firm? Red and ripe or not fully mature? Buying tomatoes that are not fully ripe is a good idea for the client who will not eat them quickly because they will ripen on the counter over a few days.

Potato: What kind? (sweet, baking, red, or gold) How large? Should you purchase an individual potato or five-pound bag?

Bread: Wheat, white, rye, sourdough, multigrain, or other? Commercial brand or freshly baked? How many loaves? It may be important to know the type of bread because of diet restrictions. Some diets restrict seeds found in multigrain breads and the amount of sugar and carbohydrates may be less in a wheat bread than white, which should be considered for the diabetic diet.

Soft drinks: Consider clear soda pop versus colas as well as diet or sugar-free and caffeinated or caffeine-free. Cans are more manageable than two liters because they are not as heavy. Another modern convenience is 6-ounce instead of 12-ounce cans of soft drinks. Ask if it is helpful to loosen or open the top (consider this on all products that have tight lids). Do not forget to ask the quantity for purchase.

Milk: Whole, two percent, one percent, fat-free, or buttermilk? A pint, quart, half gallon, or whole gallon? Again, ask if it is helpful to open the container.

Orange Juice: Frozen concentrate or already prepared? A particular brand? Acidity and high-pulp orange juice can irritate the throat and stomach, so ask if these are sensitivities.

Coffee: Is brand important? Caffeinated or not? Flavored or regular? Quantity? Ground or whole bean?

There are many options and alternatives to even a basic shopping list of milk, juice, coffee, and bread. Product packaging is another consideration. Does the client have difficulty opening certain types of packaging, such as bottle tops on beverages or the vacuum-sealed bags of potato chips? Is the client able to use a can opener or should the companion open such items? For some, squeezable bottles of condiments (i.e., ketchup, mustard, mayonnaise) may be more difficult to use because they require sufficient hand strength. Based on experience, care recipients are better able to manage smaller and lighter weight packages. This is especially important when choosing liquid products, such as beverages and laundry or dish soaps. With all the modern day choices, conveniences, and special packaging, there is really a lot to think about when going to the grocery store. A quality companion care provider is thoughtful and aware of alternatives that relate to client preferences, dietary needs, and physical abilities.

Recipes

It will be assumed that a care provider knows how to prepare boxed or frozen foods and basic recipes, such as spaghetti or macaroni and cheese. The following recipes are suggestions for simple though nutritious meals that care recipients can help prepare. Involve the care recipient as he or she is able, always considering his or her abilities and safety issues. It is a good practice to always supervise a care recipient who is using sharp objects or when near a hot stove or oven. Do not leave the kitchen in case there is an emergency.

Adapt the recipes as needed to meet dietary needs. The smaller serving-size recipes may be doubled or the larger serving-size recipes halved. It may be beneficial to make extra servings in order to have leftovers that can remain in the refrigerator for a few days or kept frozen to have in following weeks. Ask clients and family members if there are foods that are known to cause allergic reactions.

Tuna or Chicken Salad

(makes 2 servings)
6-ounce can of tuna, in water (may also use canned or cooked chicken)
½ cup mayonnaise or plain yogurt (more or less to taste)
Small squirt of mustard (any variety)
Possible additions: diced onion, celery, carrot, relish, and hard-boiled egg

Drain tuna, put in medium-size mixing bowl. Add mayonnaise or yogurt and mustard; mix well. Add other ingredients one tablespoon at a time for desired taste. Serve with or without bread.

Note: Low-fat mayonnaise or sandwich spread can be used. If a client is diabetic, consider using one slice of bread; whole wheat or multigrain is better than white bread.

Client participation: stir ingredients in mixing bowl, peel carrot, chop vegetables and egg.

Egg Salad

(makes 2 servings)
2 hard-boiled eggs
¼ cup mayonnaise or plain yogurt
1 Tablespoon yellow mustard
Salt and pepper to taste
Possible additions: relish, onion

Cover eggs with water in small saucepan and boil for 15 minutes. Rinse under cold water until eggs cool; peel. Finely chop eggs, put in medium-size mixing bowl. Add mayonnaise and mustard; stir well. Add other ingredients to preferred taste. Serve with or without bread.

Note: Low-fat mayonnaise and a salt substitute can be used. If a client is diabetic, consider using one slice of bread; whole wheat or multigrain is better than white bread.

Client participation: peel eggs (when cool), chop eggs or onion, stir ingredients.

Chicken Parmesan

(makes 1 serving)
1 uncooked chicken breast, thawed
1 egg
½–¾ cup bread crumbs
1 cup spaghetti sauce
½ cup mozzarella cheese

Heat oven to 350 degrees. Dip chicken breast in egg, and then cover with bread crumbs. Place chicken in hot, oiled skillet. Cook 2–3 minutes on each side. Place fried chicken breast in small baking dish; cover with spaghetti sauce and mozzarella cheese. Bake for 30 minutes.

Option: Chicken can be served over cooked pasta if desired. Cook pasta according to package directions. Place chicken breast on top of pasta to bake.

Note: Pre-packaged, frozen chicken breasts are a time-saving measure. To minimize carbohydrates, cooked rice can be substituted for the cooked pasta.

Client participation: dip breast in egg and bread crumbs, prepare chicken for baking by pouring sauce and placing cheese on chicken breast.

Vegetable Pasta Primavera

(makes 8 servings)
1 pound uncooked pasta
¼ cup olive oil
1½ cups broccoli florets
1½ cups sliced carrots
1 cup sliced celery

1½ cups onions (diced or in wedges)
1½ cups cauliflower
1 cup peas
Ingredients for White Sauce:
4 cups water
4 vegetable bouillon cubes or vegetable soup broth
1½ cups low-fat milk
4 rounded Tablespoons cornstarch

Cook pasta according to package directions. Drain. Combine white sauce ingredients and cook in saucepan on medium heat, being careful not to boil or scorch milk. Stir until thickened. In large skillet, sauté vegetables in oil until al dente (not cooked until soft or overdone, some firmness in the bite). Pour white sauce over vegetables in skillet, turn off heat. Place pasta on plate with vegetables and sauce on top.

Note: Fresh, frozen, or canned vegetables may be used. Chicken stock may be substituted for vegetable bouillon or broth. Vitamin D whole milk may be substituted for low fat for clients who are not on a restricted diet and may be trying to gain weight. If a client is diabetic, consider using more vegetables with whole-wheat pasta or a smaller portion of pasta.

Client participation: cut fresh vegetables if using; measure ingredients of white sauce and stir. (The care provider should consider safety concerns.)

Vegetable Soup

(makes 6–8 servings)
4 cups water
4 tablespoons vegetable, chicken, or beef bouillon
½ teaspoon oregano
¼ teaspoon pepper
1 bay leaf (optional; if using, be sure to remove from soup before serving)
1½ cups chopped tomatoes or one 14½-ounce can
½ cup peeled and cubed potatoes
10 ounces frozen corn
½ cup green beans
½ cup sliced carrots (about 2)
½ cup diced onion
15½-ounce can of kidney beans, rinsed (optional)

Bring water to a boil; add bouillon and stir until dissolved. Or, use 4 cups of canned or frozen vegetable, chicken, or beef broth. Add vegetables. Bring to a boil again, reduce heat and simmer for 30 minutes. Add kidney beans if using. Season with salt and pepper.

Note: Fresh, frozen, or canned vegetables may be used; amounts can vary depending on dietary needs, taste and preference. Low-sodium canned broths are available; use as a substitute for clients on a low-salt diet. A half pound of ground turkey or beef can be added; brown meat in another skillet before adding to the broth. Kidney beans can be used in addition or in place of a meat.

Client participation: cut tomatoes, potatoes, carrots, and onion; snap green beans (if using fresh); rinse kidney beans if using; add seasonings; measure ingredients.

Stuffed Green Pepper Soup

(makes 2–4 servings)
½ pound lean ground beef or turkey
2 teaspoons chili powder (more or less to taste)
1 cup chopped green pepper (can substitute frozen for fresh)
¼ cup diced onion
28-ounce can diced tomatoes
1 cup chicken or beef broth
½ cup white or brown rice or quick-cooking barley

Brown meat in a two-quart saucepan. Stir in chili powder; add onion, green pepper, tomatoes, and broth. Mix well. Add broth and rice or barley. Allow soup to simmer long enough to cook rice or barley if using uncooked. If already cooked, allow to simmer long enough to blend flavors.

Note: Other ingredients can be added based on client preferences while ingredients that client dislikes can be eliminated. Consider using low-sodium tomatoes and broth. Brown rice and barley have more fiber and protein than white rice.

Client participation: chop onion and green peppers; after meat is browned, mix ingredients in soup pot before returning to stovetop.

A common food intolerance is with the acids of citrus fruits, tomatoes, and tomato sauces, which may create problems with acid reflux and Gastro Esophageal Reflux Disease (GERD). To minimize symptoms, not eating spicy or acid-rich foods is recommended. The pizza recipe below is suggested for just this diet.

Tomato-Free Pizza

(Makes 2–4 servings)
One 10- or 12-inch prepared pizza crust
4 eggs
1 cup shredded Swiss cheese

In small mixing bowl, beat the eggs. Add a splash of water to thin slightly. Place pizza crust on pizza stone or baking sheet. Pour eggs over crust. Scatter cheese across the eggs. Bake pizza in oven according to package directions on crust.

Note: This is ideal for breakfast. If eating acid-rich foods do not cause a problem, add tomatoes; green peppers, onions, and other vegetables can be added if they fit into any diet restrictions.

Client participation: break and beat eggs, chop vegetables if using.

Taste buds change as people age, usually becoming duller. Many assisted living and long-term-care facilities prepare bland foods to meet the varied resident needs, especially if they house a large number of people. This can cause problems with eating and eating habits, and therefore nutrition. Residents may add salt to enhance flavor, which is not a healthy way to flavor food. The same approach is taken by older adults in their own homes. Rather than using alternative herbs and seasonings to add flavor, salt is regularly used. With creativity and the willingness to try new foods, older adults living independently have more options. Salt substitutes or herbs and spices are a healthy approach to make foods more pleasing and exciting. Food allergies and intolerance to certain types of foods can occur with age. These recipes make good use of seasonings for those who are able to tolerate spicy foods and who are looking for flavor alternatives from salt. They are also easy introductions to vegetarian and culturally sensitive cooking.

Paki-Beef

(Makes 4 servings)
1 pound lean ground beef or turkey
1 small onion, diced
1 medium carrot, sliced
10 ounces frozen spinach
2 Tablespoons (or to taste) of garam masala (or, 1 teaspoon each of: black pepper, cardamom, cumin, ginger, ground cloves)

Cook spinach on stovetop according to package directions. In another pot, brown meat; add spices. When meat is browned, add onion, carrot, and cooked spinach. Simmer for 15 minutes or until flavors are combined.

Note: Garam masala is an Indian spice blend and can be found at the grocery store.

Client participation: if using individual seasonings, measure into bowl before adding to meat; cut onion and carrots. This recipe is quick and easy to prepare.

Red Beans and Rice

(Makes 4 servings)
1 cup long-grain brown rice
2½ cups hot water
2 Tablespoons olive oil
1 medium yellow onion, diced
1 green bell pepper, seeded and diced
1 red bell pepper, seeded and diced
4 garlic cloves, minced
½ teaspoon cayenne (or red) pepper
¼ teaspoon cumin
¼ teaspoon oregano
½ teaspoon black pepper
½ teaspoon paprika
15½ ounces (1 can) kidney beans
Optional: 12 ounces fully cooked Italian or turkey sausages

In small saucepan, combine rice and water; bring to a boil. Cover, reduce to simmer, and cook for 25 minutes. After the rice has cooked for 15 minutes, heat oil in a large skillet over medium-high heat. Add onion, green and red peppers, garlic, cayenne, cumin, oregano, pepper, and paprika. Sauté and stir until onions are tender (3–5 minutes); if using sausage, add here and sauté another 3 minutes. Drain and rinse kidney beans, then add to skillet. Add the rice and remaining water in the pan. Mix well. Cover, reduce heat to medium low, and cook 5 minutes.

Note: If needed, cook sausages according to package directions before starting preparation for this recipe. It is a vegetarian recipe without adding meat.

Client participation: cut vegetables, measure spices into a separate bowl before adding to the skillet, drain and rinse beans.

Curry in a Hurry

(Makes 4 servings)
2 teaspoons curry powder
⅓ cup chicken broth
⅓ cup coconut milk
2 cups cooked boneless, skinless chicken pieces
Chopped cilantro or minced scallion (garnish)

In 2-quart saucepan over medium-high heat, whisk together curry powder, broth, and coconut milk until combined. Bring to a boil. Stir in cooked chicken pieces. Reduce heat to medium and simmer for 5 minutes. Serve over steamed rice. Add garnish.

Note: Coconut milk contains a fair amount of fat; consider using a light variety. Another alternative is to add 1 Tablespoon of coconut extract to 1 cup of low-fat milk. Already-cooked chicken pieces can be purchased. A 10-ounce package works in this recipe. If serving with rice, cook rice according to package directions.

Client participation: measure ingredients, cut chicken into small pieces.

Peanut Butter Noodles

(Makes 4 servings)
8 ounces pasta (spaghetti-size noodle works best)
½ cup creamy peanut butter
½ cup warm water
1 Tablespoon maple syrup
1 Tablespoon soy sauce
¼ teaspoon ground ginger
¼ cup scallions

Cook pasta according to package directions. Combine other ingredients in a bowl, except scallions; whisk until smooth. Drain pasta, toss with sauce. Sprinkle scallions.

Note: Soy sauce contains a large amount of salt; consider using a low-sodium variety. For easier eating, break spaghetti noodles into smaller pieces before cooking or use other small noodle. This recipe is easy to assemble and does not take much preparation time.

Client participation: measure ingredients, stir peanut sauce.

Italian Tofu and Spinach Patties (*Cooking Light Magazine,* 1986)

(Makes 4 servings)
1 pound soft tofu, drained of excess water and crumbled
10 ounces frozen, chopped spinach; thawed and squeezed dry
¼ cup parmesan cheese
1 cup shredded mozzarella cheese
½ teaspoon nutmeg
2 cloves mashed garlic
1 teaspoon salt
½ teaspoon black pepper
2 cups bread crumbs
3 Tablespoons olive oil
2 cups (or more to taste) marinara or spaghetti sauce

Mix together tofu, spinach, cheeses, nutmeg, garlic, salt, and pepper in a medium bowl. Shape mixture into 8 equal patties. Cover each patty with bread crumbs. In medium frying pan, heat oil. Sauté patties until golden on each side, about 3 minutes per side. Serve on plate, cover with marinara sauce.

Note: There are a variety of tofu types; soft (versus firm) works better in this recipe.

Client participation: measure ingredients, shred cheese, dip patties into bread crumbs. For an additional tactile activity, encourage a client to use his or her hands when mixing together ingredients. Be sure that hands are clean!

There could be clients who may or may not have diet restrictions and need to gain weight. Weight loss is a symptom of Alzheimer's and some cancers; maintaining or gaining weight may be recommended. Cheese, yogurt, ice cream, chicken or turkey pot pies, vegetarian pizza, and chili (made with ground beef or turkey) are possible suggestions for this circumstance, depending on diet restrictions. Use condiments to add calories and flavor: add butter and sour cream to casseroles and potato dishes, mayonnaise to sandwiches and fish fillets, or salad dressings to cooked vegetables and salads. Add sugar to fruits, cereals, water, tea, and coffee if that helps a client consume foods and fluids.

Quick Cooking and Planning

There may be situations when the client needs to eat quickly or to have already-prepared foods for a later time. It may be helpful to keep precut fruits and vegetables in the refrigerator for clients who eat them. Most vegetables will last longer if they are covered with water. Other healthy snacks to have available are: milk (even chocolate), cheese, crackers, peanut butter, cottage cheese, yogurt (not the "light" varieties), hard-boiled eggs, prepared pudding and Jell-O, nuts, dried fruits, olives, and pickles. Be sure these foods comply with an individual's diet restrictions.

Rice and pasta are excellent staples to have accessible for unplanned, last-minute meals. They are relatively quick and easy to cook, and there are plenty of ingredients that can be added to create a substantial meal. A quick pasta salad can be made by chopping onion and green pepper into cooked pasta and topping with low-fat bottled Italian salad dressing. Low-fat mayonnaise or plain yogurt can be used for a creamy macaroni salad. For the client who may need to gain weight, use regular mayonnaise or salad dressing. Frozen vegetables, such as broccoli or any vegetable mix, can be added to cooked pasta or rice and served hot or cold. The same vegetables can also be added to a chicken or beef broth for a quick soup or stew. Some warm foods may taste just as well cold and vice versa. For example, tuna salad can be served hot, as a casserole, with a few ingredient changes. Sandwiches can be prepared in advance if wrapped tightly and stored in the refrigerator. Ask for client ideas and preferences. Be creative with the foods on hand and suggest that these ingredients be kept readily available for quick meals.

Summary

As we age, the body may need less amounts of food though the body still requires sufficient nutrients from food. A healthy diet in aging years can reduce the risk of heart disease, high blood pressure, certain cancers, and other medical conditions. The U.S. Department of Agriculture regularly updates the Food Guide Pyramid, the guidelines of recommended food group servings for a healthy, well-balanced diet. Eating a variety of healthy foods and limiting sodium, sugar, and saturated fats from the diet will improve health.

Care recipients may be placed on special diets to meet individual needs. As the result of neurological damage, care recipients with swallowing difficulties may be placed on therapeutic diets: mechanical-soft, pureed, and thickened liquids. Other special diets are designed to restrict sodium, sugar, and carbohydrates for people with diabetes or heart-related conditions. A care provider should be fully aware of any and all diet restrictions, and only offer foods and beverages that are acceptable to the special diet. This also includes diets of preference and cultural choices—vegetarian and Kosher, for example. In addition, consider other ethnic cuisine choices. A care provider who understands the likes and dislikes of the care recipient will build better relationships and provide personalized, quality care.

Encourage care recipients to participate in meal planning and preparation. Care recipients' involvement is an opportunity for purposeful activity and stimulation; additionally, the sense of purpose contributes to their psychological well-being. Persuade the care recipient to become involved with meal planning and preparation, and to perform related tasks as independently as possible. Meal planning and preparation is an Instrumental Activity of Daily Living (IADL) that supports decision making and promotes self-sufficiency; eating or being fed is an Activity of Daily Living (ADL). These efforts are intended to keep a care recipient living independently longer.

Questions

What is meant by an "informed decision"?

Why is it important to involve the client in meal preparation?

What does the Food Guide Pyramid offer?

Name three signs of inadequate nutrition in an older person.

How is a pleasant dining experience significant to a care recipient's well-being?

How can a care provider contribute to a positive dining experience?

What is the number one rule of meal preparation?

Explain the differences between mechanical-soft and pureed diets.

When is a thickened liquid diet appropriate?

What foods are not acceptable to a diabetic diet? A low-sodium diet?

Summary Tips

Have a general idea of what foods are considered nutritious and encourage a care recipient to eat as many of these foods as the care recipient is willing.

Be familiar with the USDA's Food Guide Pyramid.

Understand the various therapeutic and cultural diets by knowing what foods are and are not acceptable to the diet and to clients' preferences.

To encourage independence and decision making, persuade care recipients' participation in meal planning and preparation.

Helpful Web Sites

Diabetic Diets: http://www.nlm.nih.gov/medlineplus/diabeticdiet.html

Food and Public Policy: U.S. Department of Agriculture at http://www.usda.gov

Education for food and nutrition professionals: American Dietetics Association at http://www.eatright.org

Food and Drug Administration: http://www.fda.gov

Kosher Dietary laws: Judaism 101 at http://www.jewfaq.org

U.S. Department of Agriculture: http://www.usda.gov

Vegetarian diets and recipes: http://www.vegetarianrecipesite.com

Suggested Reading

Adderly, Brenda, & De Angelis, Lissa. (2004). *The arthritis cure cookbook*. New York: St. Martin's Press. More than 100 recipes to help alleviate arthritis pain, boost antioxidants, and rebuild damaged joints.

Balch, Phyllis. (2006). *Prescription for nutritional healing*. New York: Penguin Group. Provides drug-free alternatives using vitamins, minerals, herbs, and food supplements.

Blumenthal, Roger, & Hermanson, Juli. (2004). *Betty Crocker's healthy heart cookbook*. Hoboken, NJ: John Wiley and Sons. Heart-healthy recipes, menu planning, nutritional analysis, and health resource guide.

Eugene, Linda, Spitler, Sue, & Yoakam, Linda (Eds.). (2007). *1001 delicious recipes for people with diabetes* (2nd ed.). Chicago: Surrey Books. Recipes based on the latest recommendations for the diabetic diet, including nutritional analysis, diabetic food exchanges, monitoring carbohydrate intake, and exercise for the diabetic person.

Katzen, Mollie. (2000). *The enchanted broccoli forest*. Berkeley, CA: Ten Speed Press. Easy-to-prepare vegetarian dishes and meals, plus tips and techniques in the kitchen.

Rombauer, Irma, Rombauer Becker, Marion, & Becker, Ethan. (2006). *The joy of cooking 75th anniversary edition*. New York: Scribner. Four thousand recipes, nutritional information, tips for storing food, and meal planning.

Home Safety and Household Management

10

In This Chapter, You Will Learn

1. To recognize responsibilities for keeping the home safe, and ways to increase safety

2. How to use creativity and problem-solving skills to make the home safer

3. Medical equipment and supplies common in the home care environment

4. The concept and use of Universal Design

Why This Matters

Issues of safety are a significant concern and the major reason that home care recipients are placed in a supervised living environment, such as an assisted living or long-term-care facility. To keep a care recipient safe in the home is to prevent them from physical injury, environmental hazards, medication inaccuracies, and certain social influences. Home safety encompasses anything from the supervision of daily medication routines and meal intake, to ensuring that a working fire extinguisher is available, to arranging for adaptive home medical equipment. Protecting the home care recipient can mean monitoring phone calls from dishonest sales promotions and keeping floors clear of clutter to prevent falls. Maintaining safety in the home may make the difference between the care recipient staying in the home or needing to move into a long-term-care facility. The goal of home care is to keep care recipients living at home for as long as possible. It is the role and responsibility of a home care provider to ensure a safe, hazard-free environment that supports independent living.

Keeping the Home Safe

A major responsibility of the care provider is to provide a safe living environment for the care recipient. This means constant supervision to prevent falls, minimize household hazards, infection control, and prepare for emergencies and natural disasters, such as winter storms. Equipment safety is also a component of household safety.

Case Study

Jacob had osteoporosis and a degenerative bone condition that caused him to fall frequently. His apartment was small and the walls created a maze-like hallway. He was unsteady on his feet and had difficulty maintaining his balance. Jacob pushed his walker through the sharp turns of the narrow hallway, walking 20 feet from the kitchen on one end of the apartment to his bedroom on the other end. He often fell while navigating around the furniture and through the narrow corridor.

Fortunately, the falls were seldom serious enough for him to get badly hurt, though he was unable to raise himself. Against everyone's advice, Jacob refused to wear a medical alarm bracelet or necklace, though he carried a cordless and cell phone with him most times. He needed another person to lift him after a fall, which required that he call his son, friends, or neighbors for assistance. The telephone numbers were near the kitchen, which meant he had to scoot himself along the floor and down the corridor to the kitchen. Most times, Jacob did not have the strength or energy to maneuver movement after falling. After a number of falls in his bedroom and several nights on the floor, he told his care provider, Robin, of the incidents and his inability to pick himself up. Looking at the problem from Jacob's point of view, Robin created a plan of action specific to his needs. She wrote Jacob's preferred contact names and numbers on four different pieces of paper and placed one list in every room. Where Robin placed the lists was key: She taped the phone number lists on the wall where it meets the floor. Robin realized that his falling may be inevitable, but if he was going to fall, he would need easy access to the phone numbers. Placing the lists at eye level would not have served the same purpose because they would not be viewable if Jacob was on the floor. Robin's creative approach was not to prevent Jacob from falling, rather to provide a practical adaptation for managing his situation.

The care provider should watch for potential problems and take necessary steps to prevent accidents from happening during regular visits with the care recipient. This can be done with or without the care recipient knowing that the care provider is assessing home safety measures. On each visit, complete a room-by-room inventory to notice obscure and obvious risks that can interfere with the care recipient's personal and home safety.

Every caregiving situation and environment is different. It is beneficial for the care provider to set up a daily, weekly, or monthly schedule to monitor home-safety issues. This is a good habit to establish, keeping in mind that emergency and safety concerns can and do happen at any time.

To determine if a condition is an issue, ask yourself if the care recipient is able to cope and accomplish daily routines. If conditions are difficult, dangerous, or unmanageable, brainstorm ideas of how the situation could be better. Then, consider how the care recipient, with compromised physical or mental functioning, could better handle the problem or emergency. Discuss with the care recipient and determine if he or she can cope with the changes in an urgent situation. Approach these conversations with respect, reminding the care recipient that his or her independence is the main goal.

Use problem-solving skills and draw on past experiences to offer care recipients resourceful ideas that create easier and more favorable conditions. For example, if the fire extinguisher is kept in the basement, move it underneath the kitchen or bathroom sink, or anywhere else that is quickly accessible to the care recipient. A yardstick or broom handle is a useful tool for turning on light switches or manipulating hard-to-reach objects when trying to make contact with something above shoulder level; if appropriate, make these adaptive tools available. Furniture may need to be rearranged or removed to make the home easier to navigate, particularly when a care recipient is in a wheelchair. A common home adaptation is to move the clothes washer and dryer from the basement to a utility or spare room on the first floor for accessibility. These supportive living adaptations encourage independent performance of Activities of Daily Living and Instrumental Activities of Daily Living.

Change is difficult. Be sensitive when altering the home, particularly if the care recipient has lived there for a number of years. Think about care recipients who have lived in their home for 30 years and can find their way around the house in the middle of the night without lights; a table moved just four inches can interfere with the care recipient's functioning when he or she remembers it in another position. Drastic changes can be upsetting and disruptive to otherwise normal routines and the adjustment process can be difficult. First discuss the adaptations with the care recipient and make sure there is agreement before making the changes; even still, it will take the care recipient time to learn and become familiar with the new arrangements.

There are some home conditions that cannot be altered. In many homes, the breaker box (needed when the power goes out) is located in the basement. What if the electricity goes out and the care recipient is physically unable to get up and down the stairs? It would be cost prohibitive to relocate the circuit board or breaker box to an upper level; other options need to be considered. A potential solution is to provide a trusted neighbor with the care recipient's house key, with permission from the care recipient and family. The neighbor may experience the same power outage and know to help the care recipient; because of proximity, it is assumed that the neighbor could get to the care recipient's home faster than others.

The following are suggestions to increase safety in the care recipient's home. The care provider should give attention to these areas, while keeping in mind other angles of personal and home safety issues.

First-Aid Kit

A good practice for care providers is to carry a personal first-aid kit, even if it is left in the car during visits. It is essential for emergency preparation. First-aid kits can be homemade or purchased already assembled. Care recipients should also keep a first-aid kit or emergency supplies accessible in the home. Personalized kits can include incidentals unique to the care recipient, such as specific medications or emergency contact information. Store the kit in an accessible but secure place, especially if the care recipient has dementia or if children could come in contact with potentially harmful substances.

A basic first-aid kit should include:

An assortment of adhesive bandages and other wraps
Medical tape
Gauze and cotton swabs
Hand cleaner, such as an alcohol-based waterless solution
Antibacterial and antiseptic ointment
Hydrogen Peroxide
Isopropyl (rubbing) alcohol
Disposable gloves
Plastic bags
Scissors, tweezers, and needles
Thermometer
Aspirin or acetaminophen
Ipecac syrup (vomit inducer)
Emergency phone number and contact list
Flashlight, with extra batteries

In addition to a first-aid kit, other needed supplies that should be accessible are:

Antibacterial ointment
Batteries (common household appliance sizes)
Compression hose
Denture care and cleaning supplies
Diabetic needle disposal container
Disposable gloves
Blankets and sheets
Gauze bandages and cotton balls

Heating pad and ice pack

Incontinence supplies (protective underwear, briefs, liners, underpads, body wipes)

Laxatives

Lotion

Rubbing alcohol and hydrogen peroxide

Supplemental drinks

Thermometer

Tissues

Toilet paper

Extra blankets come in handy—know where they are kept in care recipients' homes or store one or two in your car. A bag of frozen peas or other vegetables can be used as a cold or hot (heat in microwave) pack. Towels, sheets, sanitary napkins, and incontinence pads can be used to control heavy bleeding. Ammonia or vinegar can be applied to insect bites. Other home products can be used for comfort or in emergency situations; be creative and resourceful (see also Tip 10.1).

Tip 10.1

Tips for Emergencies

Burns

If a care recipient burns him- or herself, provide immediate care by running cold water over the affected area or by applying a cold compress to stop the burning. For a severe burn where clothing sticks to the skin, call 911 or quickly transport the care recipient to the emergency room.

Bleeding

Even minor cuts, scrapes, and skin tears can produce a large amount of blood from an older adult because of thin skin or certain medications, such as blood thinners. To assist a care recipient who is bleeding, cover the open area with a clean cloth and apply pressure. If possible, wear gloves or use anything plastic as a barrier in an effort to not have contact with the blood. Continue to place pressure on the wound until bleeding stops, adding other clean cloths on top of the blood-soaked cloth as needed. If the bleeding area is on the leg, toe, arm, or finger, elevate the extremity above the heart to decrease blood flow. The care provider should be sure to wash hands thoroughly as soon as possible to prevent the spread of infection. Call 911 if the bleeding is severe and does not stop.

Fainting (also called Syncope)

Heart problems, certain medications, low blood sugar, standing too quickly, and dehydration, which are common conditions in older adults, are known to cause a person to faint. Fainting can occur when the blood pressure suddenly drops, which decreases the flow of blood to the brain. There is a temporary loss of consciousness and muscle control that can result in the care recipient falling.

To prevent episodes of fainting:

Learn if a care recipient is on medications that can cause fainting (ask a pharmacist or doctor)

If the care recipient is on medications that cause fainting, talk with family members or other health care providers about the possibility of medication changes

Encourage or arrange for regular blood-sugar-level checks

Encourage the care recipient to hold on to something (a piece of furniture, grab bar) and to stand slowly

Promote fluids to keep the care recipient hydrated

Encourage the care recipient to sit or lie down when feeling faint

If a care recipient faints, the home care provider should:

Lay the care recipient flat on his or her back

Elevate the legs, if possible, above the heart

Check breathing and pulse; make sure the airway is clear

Monitor for any movement, including coughing

Loosen restrictive clothing

Cover the care recipient with a blanket and keep comfortable

Do not offer fluids

Begin CPR and call 911 if the care recipient does not regain consciousness within minutes

Seizures

There are different types of seizures with varying degrees of symptoms. The most commonly observed symptom is the uncontrollable shaking of the body. Seizures occur because of abnormal electrical activity in the brain, which can be caused by medications, head injuries, and certain diseases. A seizure usually lasts 30 seconds to 2 minutes; if it lasts longer than 5 minutes, call 911. When a home care recipient is having a seizure, provide the following:

Lay the care recipient flat on the floor or bed

If the care recipient is convulsing, remove objects nearby that could cause injury

Surround the care recipient with pillows and blankets for protection

Roll the care recipient on his or her side to keep the airway open

Do not restrain the care recipient; allow uncontrollable movements to happen

Do not give the care recipient food or drink until he or she is completely alert and responsive

Conduct CPR if the care recipient stops breathing or has no pulse; if breathing is not restored, call 911

Bathroom Safety

Many hazards wait in the bathrooms, which is typically smaller than other rooms in the house and can limit mobility. Walker legs and shuffling feet can become entangled on carpeted floor surfaces. There is great potential for slipping or falling on wet, uncarpeted floors. Generally, people place bathmats or other water-catching rugs on a bathroom floor; these present the opportunity for tripping over the edges and can result in a fall. Mats and throw rugs can be taped or tacked down to prevent moving if it is necessary to have them. Water temperatures can be an issue. The care provider should inform others who may oversee household maintenance to ensure that the water heater is set accordingly.

Suggestions for keeping the bathroom safe include:

Place textured or nonskid mats in the shower, bathtub, or on the bathroom floor

Install grab bars near the toilet, tub, shower, and counters for support

Make arrangements for a shower chair or handheld showerhead

Check water temperatures to make sure they are not too hot or too cold

Ensure there is appropriate lighting, adding a nightlight if needed

It may be helpful to the care recipient if the care provider sets up the bathing situation, even when not providing direct ADL care. Placing towels, toiletries (soap and shampoo), and a clean change of clothes in the bathroom can aid the independent care recipient in the bathing process.

Preventing Falls

Falls are the primary cause of injury to the elderly. Often the consequence of a fall is a change in lifestyle or the living situation. The care provider's responsibility toward home safety is one step toward keeping the care recipient living independently longer. Take precautionary measures to protect the care recipient from unnecessary harm, such as removing obstacles that interfere with easy mobility and everyday routine.

Consider these methods to prevent a fall:

Remove objects from the floor, such as shoes, newspapers, and cords

Secure (with tape or nails) or remove throw rugs

Use nonskid mats in the bathroom and kitchen

Install grab bars and handrails in necessary places

Use bedrails to prevent falling out of bed and as a measure of security while turning/rolling over during sleep times

Clear pathways around regularly used furniture (chairs, couches, tables)

Forbid foot traffic on wet floors; wipe up spills immediately

Keep areas well lit and install additional lights (i.e., nightlights)

Use higher wattage light bulbs, 60–75 watts for maximum lighting

The care recipient can contribute to fall prevention through maintenance of personal routines. Vision should be checked annually to detect deficiencies.

Care recipients can wear nonskid slippers, which are usually adequate, although a sturdy shoe that provides support is generally better. If orthopedic shoes are needed, a professional (i.e., physical therapist) should provide assistance. Encourage the care recipient to be aware and move with caution, particularly if he or she is recuperating from a fall. Regular exercise can maintain or improve strength and coordination. The care recipient may benefit from a walking aid, such as a cane or walker. Canes are available at pharmacies and medical equipment supply outlets. A pharmacist, medical equipment representative, or physical or occupational therapist should demonstrate the correct way to use a cane. There are many styles and varieties of available walkers: no wheels, two wheels, or four wheels. The best-practice judgment is to have a physical therapist or nurse evaluate the care recipient to determine what medical equipment meets his or her needs (see also Tip 10.2).

Tip 10.2

Managing Visual and Auditory Impairments

Visual Aids

Prescription eyeglasses
Magnifying glasses and sheets
Large-print texts
Books on tape or compact discs
Additional and brighter lighting

Hearing Devices

Prescribed hearing aids
Amplification systems, including microphones and telephone amplifiers
Close-captioned television

Medical Equipment and Supply Safety

Initially, physical and occupational therapists should perform in-home evaluations to determine the best-suited equipment for the home care client. Physical and occupational therapists, nurses, pharmacists, and medical equipment representatives may train the home care provider on correct methods of use and recommendations on how to assist the care recipient with adaptive devices and equipment. The home care provider should have an understanding of the goal and function of the care recipient's medical equipment. Even if the care recipient applies the apparatus, it may become a responsibility of the home care provider to monitor and observe that equipment is used appropriately for maximum effectiveness. Instruction manuals are almost always provided with a new product. Most equipment is adjustable and adaptable to individual needs. A list of commonly used special and adaptive equipment used in the home caregiving situation is listed below.

Mobility aids help a person move, transfer, or walk. They include the following:

Wheelchair: allows the care recipient using it to propel the self or to be pushed from behind by another person. Remove the foot pedals from the wheelchair and be sure to secure the brakes when the care recipient is transferring in and out of the chair.

Walker (with or without wheels, see Figure 10.1): provides support to maintain balance and can provide a sense of safety to the care recipient. Make sure the walker "clicks" when in the open position. A care recipient may need to be evaluated by a physical therapist periodically to be sure that the walker is safe and appropriate to the care recipient's functioning level.

10.1

Two-wheeled walker

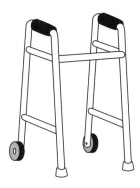

Cane (straight or quad, with four prongs): provides light weight-bearing support. Canes have very specific functions and different cane types have special purposes. To be sure the cane is being used correctly, discuss proper use with the care recipient, physical therapist, nurse, or pharmacist. A straight cane and quad cane are pictured in Figure 10.2.

10.2

Quad cane, straight cane

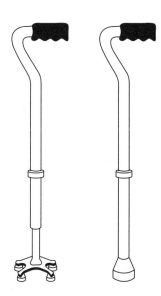

Electric Scooter (three or four wheels): operated with a joystick by the person using it.

To minimize accidents and hazards, the care recipient using an electric scooter should move at minimal speeds, especially when in crowds. If the scooter is operated on public sidewalks and streets, make certain that the scooter is very visible to automobile traffic.

Many scooter drivers attach a 6-foot-tall orange or red flag to the chair so that it can be seen from a distance, as seen in Figure 10.3.

10.3

Motorized scooter (3 wheel)

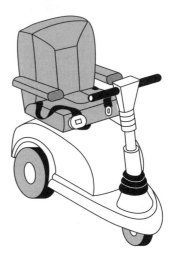

Gait belt: placed around the waist to support a care recipient's balance (see Figure 10.4). It is used by the person providing assistance. Because gait belts should be used as support, they are unsafe for use on an immobile care recipient and should not be the means for lifting or holding up a person.

10.4

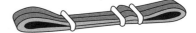

Gait belt

Transfer board (in varying lengths): One end is placed where the care recipient is sitting to prepare for the transfer; the other end rests on the place where the care recipient is moving. Typically used when transferring from the wheelchair to couch, bed, or toilet.

The care recipient will scoot him- or herself across the board to transfer from one place of sitting to another. It can be used independently by the home care client or the care provider can offer assistance. If the care recipient uses the board independently, see that proper training has been provided. Home care providers should also be trained on the proper use of a transfer board.

Bedroom equipment and supplies range from items of comfort to assistive devices that aid mobility to large equipment. Common bedroom equipment and supplies are listed below.

Hospital bed: offers better positioning options for comfort and good skin care to prevent pressure sores. The ability to move the bed up and down electrically can make transferring in and out of bed easier.

Bed rails: attach to the side of the bed and prevent a care recipient from rolling out of bed. The rails should be lowered when getting out of bed and in the up position while the person is sleeping. Most rails are not durable enough to use as a transfer aid, including raising oneself out of bed (see Figure 10.5).

10.5

Hospital bed with rails

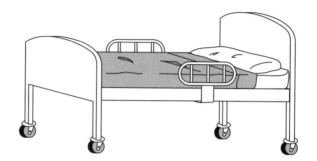

Air mattress: An electric pump fills a mattress with air to reduce pressure against the skin. The air pressure can be adjusted to meet individual needs.

Egg carton pad: shaped like an egg carton, this foam mattress pad is placed underneath the fitted sheet. These pads promote air circulation beneath the body and can minimize pressure between the bed and body. They are often used to prevent bedsores.

Bed cane: used to transfer in and out of bed. It is a triangular handrail affixed upright to a square board or rectangular metal tubing that slides between the box springs and mattress. Figure 10.6 shows how the board or tubing slides under the mattress. Similar to a walking cane, it provides support to maintain balance when standing or sitting.

10.6

Couch/bed cane

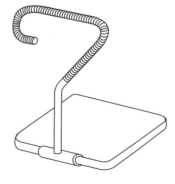

Trapeze bar: The triangular steel bar hangs over the bed and is attached to a large apparatus that is securely installed at the head of the bed (see Figure 10.7). The adjustable trapeze is used for rising up, changing positions, and transferring in and out of bed.

10.7

Trapeze bar

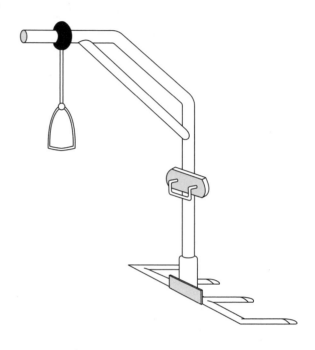

Hoyer Hydraulic Lift: a large steel apparatus with a cloth (usually canvas) cradle in which a care recipient sits for transferring (see Figure 10.8). This piece of equipment is practical for heavy and difficult-to-move people. To prevent falls and other hazards, be sure the person who is being transferred is sitting correctly in the cradle.

10.8

Hoyer hydraulic lift

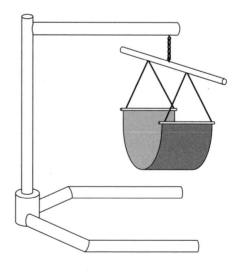

Bed wedges: variously shaped foam pillows used for positioning. They may be used to elevate feet, legs, neck, and back.

Blanket support: elevates blankets off of the body, especially the feet, to minimize pressure on the skin. The metal tubing is inserted between the box springs and mattress.

Bed pads (also known as chuck, incontinence, or under pads): disposable or reusable pads that lay on top of the fitted sheet to protect the mattress and sheets from getting wet. Pads can also be placed on furniture (chairs, couches) for protection as well as the seat of a wheelchair.

Portable commode (or bedside commode): usually placed in the bedroom for toileting ease during the night (see Figure 10.9).The pail that catches the urine or bowel movements lifts easily from the chair and the contents can be dumped into the toilet. Portable or bedside commodes are ideal for home care clients with limited mobility or who have the urgent need to use the bathroom.

10.9

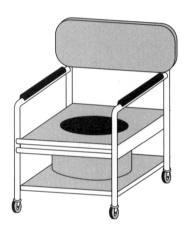

Portable commode (or bedside commode)

Urinal or bed pan: a container for catching urine while lying in bed. Typically, they are made out of a heavy-duty plastic. Specific designs for use by men and women are available (see Figure 10.10).

10.10

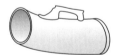

Male urinal

Devices are available to assist with dressing. Some of these tools can be difficult to use, especially if the home care recipient has limited use with one or both hands and arms. Buttonhooks, to make buttoning shirts and pants easier, may be helpful. Sock aids and shoehorns can be useful for the care recipient who has difficulty bending over to pull up socks and put on shoes. Physical and occupational therapists should be consulted to make evaluations for proper equipment and can offer training to the care recipient and care provider.

Bathroom equipment and supplies are plentiful and as diverse as the need.

Bath bench: a bench in varying lengths that is placed in the shower or bathtub. The bench provides a place to sit while showering that is not as low as sitting in the bathtub, which aids those who have difficulty moving up and down from the tub (see Figure 10.11). Be sure rubber stoppers are on the bottom of each bench leg to prevent sliding and tipping.

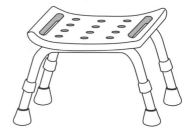

10.11

Bath bench

Shower seat: a seat that is fixed to the shower wall or transportable. Very similar to a bath bench, it provides a place to sit when showering. If the seat is not permanently attached, be sure the chair is securely placed to prevent tipping.

Transfer bench: assists a care recipient with moving in and out of the bathtub and provides a place to sit while bathing. Two of the four legs are on the outside of the tub while the other two legs are on the inside, making it easier for the care recipient using it to sit on the bench and slide across. Figure 10.12 shows how the bench is correctly placed.

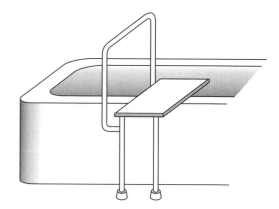

10.12

Transfer bench

Handheld shower: a portable showerhead with a long hose (see Figure 10.13). This makes it possible for the care recipient to manage the direction of water flow while sitting on a shower chair or bench.

10.13

Handheld shower

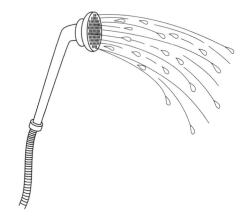

Rubber bath mat: Suction cups on the bottom of the mat secure it to the bathtub or shower floor to prevent slipping and falling. A rubber bathmat should be placed in the tub or shower for the home care client who stands in the shower and does not use a shower seat or bench.

Long-handled sponge: A foam sponge is on one end of the long handle for cleaning hard-to-reach places on the body. This utensil is ideal for a care recipient who is unable to bend over or reach difficult places, such as toes, ankles, and the back.

Raised toilet seat: The elevated seat makes it easier to stand up or sit down on the toilet seat. They are made from a heavy-duty plastic and are tightly secured to the toilet to prevent movement.

Toilet safety frame: provides assistance with sitting down and standing up from the toilet (see Figure 10.14). Similar to bed canes, the handles on both sides of the toilet offer support to maintain balance when standing or sitting.

10.14

Toilet safety frame

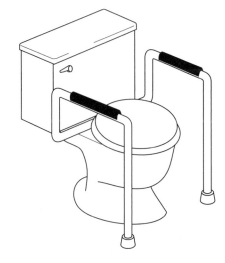

Grab or safety bar: steel bars of varying lengths can be placed in the tub and shower to assist with getting in and out of the shower or tub. Figure 10.15 shows grab bars, which are often found in the bathroom and next to a toilet to assist with moving on and off the toilet. Bars should be sturdy enough to hold the weight of the person using them; they provide support and help the care recipient maintain balance.

10.15

Grab bars

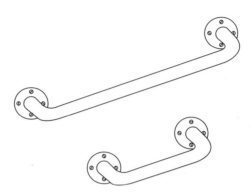

Around the house equipment and supplies include helpful gadgets and aids used in the kitchen and common areas.

Can opener (electric): When attached to the wall or other sturdy surface, the care recipient with limited use of one or both hands can more easily operate the opener while holding the can.

Plate guard: a movable device that provides an edge to any side of a plate. By placing the guard on the plate, a care recipient with limited hand or arm mobility can more easily move food onto a fork or spoon.

Swivel spoon: The bowl-end of the spoon is curved in a perpendicular position from the handle, creating direct and easy access to the mouth. This tool is helpful for those who have limited hand and wrist mobility. Foam added to utensil handles that increases thickness can be more manageable. An occupational therapist will make recommendations for these adaptations.

Lazy Susan: a rotating round tray for storing items. This can be placed on a counter or table with regularly used items for easy access; consider using a Lazy Susan that has two or three shelves.

Lift chair: These motorized easy chairs rise from the back to enable the care recipient to reach an almost-standing position (see Figure 10.16). Lift chairs are advantageous for those who have difficulty moving up and down from a seated position. Each chair has an attached foot rest that opens when the chair is in the recline position.

Couch cane: Comparable to the bed cane, couch canes provide assistance with maintaining balance when standing and sitting from a couch or chair. The cane is secured underneath the couch to offer maximum support when the care recipient bears weight during use (see Figure 10.6).

10.16

Lift chair

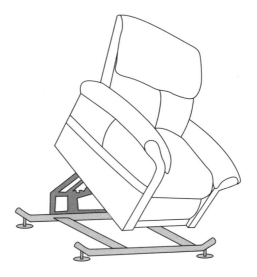

Pillows and cushions: add comfort, support, and elevation when standing is difficult.

Pillows or cushions can be set on chairs and couches, car and wheelchair seats, or used on the bed for positioning.

Grabber/Reacher: used to pick up small and lightweight objects (see Figure 10.17). There are a variety of types and styles that can be used in various ways. Grabbers and reachers are multipurpose tools. With good manipulation, they can be used to pick up paper and clothes and helpful with pulling on socks or moving a plate of food. Encourage a care recipient to keep a grabber or reacher in each room or to carry one with them at all times, even when leaving home.

10.17

Grabbers/reachers

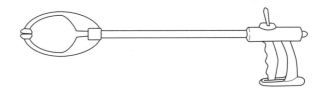

Grab ropes: attach cords to bed posts made from rope, towels, sheets, or bathrobe sashes for use when changing positions or moving in and out of bed.

Ramp: makes getting through doorways or over elevated surfaces easier for clients in wheelchairs. The more common ramps are those for loading a wheelchair into a van or ramps from a driveway (or the outdoors) to the front door; just as essential are ramps inside the home (see Figure 10.18). Threshold ramps are designed for placement in doorways and over raised surfaces. These ramps create a smooth slope over uneven and angled surfaces for easier mobility.

Stair lift: transports the care recipient up and down stairs by way of a permanent, motorized chair. The lift can be installed on either side of the staircase, though needs to be attached to a wall, not the handrail. Figure 10.19 shows a

10.18

Ramp

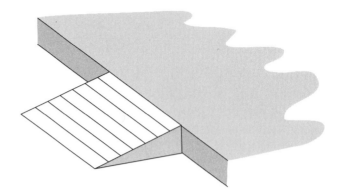

10.19

Stair lift

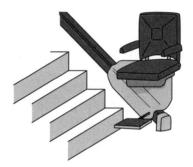

stair lift. The seat may swivel; be sure the care recipient is properly secured in the seat before operating the lift.

Emergency response button: a wrist or necklace medallion that quickly connects to the local fire department for emergency services when the button is activated. Encourage home care recipients to wear the alert button at all times. Additionally, the emergency response system should be placed in a central location in the living space so that the care recipient can hear the instructions from the emergency respondent. This equipment is tested regularly by the emergency response service provider; assist the care recipient with ensuring the equipment is working effectively.

Brace (for ankles, legs, arms, or back): there are several varieties with specific functions and purpose. The care recipient and the home care provider should be trained on applying the apparatus correctly by a physical or occupational therapist or nurse.

Oxygen tank: allows for easier breathing, though is not a tool for artificial breathing.

Oxygen tanks can be very hazardous. There are necessary precautions that must be taken to avoid danger. Oxygen is flammable: Keep tanks away from flames, high heat, aerosols, alcohol, cigarettes, gasoline, and perfume. Tanks should be stored in a stable, upright position and should not lie on their side.

A home care provider should not suggest medical guidance related to oxygen levels, which should be regulated and monitored by a medical professional. Difficulties with operating the equipment should be directed to the medical equipment representative. Follow instructions provided by the oxygen supplier and make contact names and phone numbers accessible.

Home infusion equipment: administers intravenous antibiotics, chemotherapy, pain management, and nutrition treatments. This type of equipment is used with severe diabetic, cancer, and AIDS patients.

Fire Safety

Fire prevention is best presented as guidelines for safety.

Install smoke detectors. Batteries need to be checked at least once a year and changed as needed. For maximum protection, place at least one smoke detector on each floor.

Test the alarm on each floor to be sure the siren warnings can be heard throughout the entire level.

Smoking is a major risk for home fires. The best method of prevention is not allowing an unsafe care recipient to smoke unsupervised, though this may require intervention from family members. Do not allow a care recipient to smoke in bed and recommend that the care recipient smoke in only one room to eliminate further risk. Never let the care recipient smoke near an oxygen tank!

Post emergency numbers near all telephones, including 911. In an emergency, it may be hard for the care recipient to think clearly and to remember 911. It is an extra measure of security to have this number posted.

Discourage the use of fireplaces. If that is the primary heat source, make sure it is cleaned out seasonally and that only wood, not paper, is burned.

Position space heaters at least 3 feet away from all furniture, wallpaper, clothing, or other flammable materials. Never leave a heater unattended or turned on when the room or house has been vacated.

When cooking on the stovetop, clear the area of anything that could catch on fire and turn the pot handles inward so they cannot be bumped off the stove. Loose clothes, such as the arms of house robes, are a hazard because they can ignite if there is close contact with a hot burner. Grease fires are extremely dangerous; adding water in an attempt to put out a grease fire is disastrous. Use a pan lid to smother the flames and turn off the burner.

Keep kitchen appliances clean. Grease and food build-up can add to machine malfunction (see also Tip 10.3).

Do not use appliances with broken or frayed electrical cords and do not overload electrical outlets or power strips. Turn off and unplug an appliance if there is an unusual smell.

A written fire-escape plan is most ideal but not always typical. In the least, discuss and review with the care recipient what should occur in the event of an emergency.

One fire extinguisher per floor is ideal. A smaller fire extinguisher may be more manageable for the care recipient, particularly if he or she has impaired physical functioning. Care providers should be trained on how to properly use an extinguisher.

Tip 10.3

Other Tips for Kitchen Safety

Place silverware handles up in the dishwasher; in case a care recipient falls onto an open dishwasher door, sharp items will not be upright.

Open hard-to-open cans, bottles, and jars; not only is this helpful, but it could prevent spills and breakage.

Pour liquids from large, heavy bottles into smaller containers that are more manageable; this can also prevent unnecessary spills.

Store foods in smaller containers for manageability; heavy pots and dishes are less controllable and are more easily dropped.

Monitor the refrigerator for old and spoiled foods; clear it out weekly or more often.

If mugs with handles are easier to manage, encourage their use.

Place nonskid rubber mats or coasters on counters and tables to prevent sliding and spills.

Tape a paint-stirring stick or yardstick (of needed length) onto the faucet to make it reachable. This is especially helpful for care recipients who are in wheelchairs and have difficulty reaching or standing up to turn on the water.

Tie shoelaces or ribbons on cabinet door handles for easy grabbing.

Infection Control

Elderly and ill people usually have weaker immune systems, making them more susceptible to viruses (i.e., cold and flu) and infections. There are specific infection control guidelines, known as Universal Precautions, that are guidelines for minimizing the spread of infection. In the medical field, Universal Precautions instruct care providers on how to avoid contact with another person's bodily fluids, including blood, urine, and saliva. A care provider should not make direct contact with these fluids and should handle any instrument that touches the care recipient's skin and fluids with extreme caution.

The best practice for preventing infection is to wash hands regularly. Hand washing should be a routine habit after touching the care recipient, pets, trash cans, and other objects that collect germs. Kitchens and bathrooms can be full of germs; use good judgment and wash your hands regularly. Encourage care recipients who receive services to also keep their hands clean and offer them assistance with hand washing if needed. People with Alzheimer's disease or dementia frequently forget to wash their hands after using the bathroom and may need direction: Demonstrate hand washing or turn on the water, put soap in the care recipient's hands, physically put their hands together to start the process.

Disposable gloves are a common practice to avoid infection, especially if there is a greater possibility of touching bodily fluids. Gloves should be used only one time and then disposed. Generally, a care provider should not perform personal care routines that require direct contact with a care recipient. A nurse or home health aide will provide these personal care procedures in needed situations. Unexpected incidents happen though, and the companion may have to clean up spills. Wear gloves to wipe up blood or urine that falls on the floor and dispose of the rags or towels. Use bleach or another cleaning agent to thoroughly clean and disinfect the affected area. It is better to be aware of precautionary measures that prevent the spread of infection; when in doubt, wear gloves to protect yourself as well as the care recipient.

Most home health agencies and organizations provide thorough training in Universal Precautions and infection control. To learn more about these preventive methods, ask the agency for detailed information.

Natural Disasters

Often there is time to prepare for hurricanes and snow, ice, and wind storms. Other natural disasters, such as tornadoes, come without much warning. There may be occasions when care providers or family members are unable to get to the care recipient's home during a disaster. It is a good practice to prepare him or her and the home situation for weather emergencies that are typical to the local area. A care recipient should be prepared to act alone in the event of a natural disaster. Neighbors may be able to offer some help, but it is better to pre-plan with emergency essentials and a disaster plan, and review this plan with the care recipient.

The American Red Cross recommends storing 3 days' worth of provisions for each person in the household to prepare for an emergency. When preparing emergency kits, assemble similar supplies found in a first-aid kit, plus items particular to the emergency event. For example, gloves, hats, and cold-weather clothing are more critical in the event of a snow or ice storm than during a hurricane.

A basic emergency supply kit may include:

Blankets and pillows
Flashlight with extra batteries
Battery-operated radio with extra batteries
First-aid kit
Basic tool kit: hammer, pliers, screwdriver, tape, plastic bags, scissors, and
    can opener
Extra cash
Clothing: extra coats, gloves, hats, and socks
Food: nonperishable foods that do not require refrigeration, cooking, or
    water (ready-to-eat foods such as peanut butter, snack bars, soups,
    canned meats)

At a minimum, one gallon of water per person per day

Personal items: extra eyeglasses, contact lens supplies, hearing-aid batteries, feminine products, and personal hygiene items

Medications: prescription names and numbers

List of important phone numbers: police, fire, pharmacy, doctor, health care providers, family members, and neighbors

Important papers: personal identification, medication lists, and insurance (i.e., Medicare) information

Miscellaneous: towels and paper towels, rags, pet supplies, books, magazines, and word puzzles

Disaster supplies and kits should be kept in an out of the way yet accessible place. A first-floor closet may be the best location so that the care recipient does not need to navigate stairs. Supplies can be placed in bags or small boxes. Lighter weight containers are more manageable than one heavy box filled with supplies. The care recipient will need to be able to reach and lift the supply kits. Remember, this preparedness is for the event that a care recipient will be home alone when disaster happens and no one is able to get to the home to assist. Regularly review with the care recipient where these supplies are stored and what procedures should take place in an emergency. It will not be productive to have the provisions in place without the care recipient knowing where the emergency supplies are kept and what to do.

The American Red Cross has emergency and disaster preparedness programs that provide information and education. Consult the local chapter for additional instruction for emergency preparation procedures specific to your area.

General Safety in the Home

There are general guidelines a care provider should think about on a regular basis in addition to the above-mentioned safety precautions. If the care recipient is unable to visit a medical supply store, the care provider could visit a store or search the Internet to get ideas for creating a safer living environment. The following suggestions are specifically for the care provider working with a home care recipient:

Place a list of emergency contact phone numbers, including 911, by each telephone.

Clean care recipients' eyeglass lenses.

If care recipient uses a hearing aid, make sure it works properly and replace batteries often.

Make sure floors, hallways, doorways, and staircases are clutter free.

Wipe up spills as they happen, using Universal Precaution methods as needed.

When appropriate, suggest an emergency response system.

Add grab bars or handrails near steps, especially in doorways. Grab bars should also be considered in the bathroom, along with a shower stool.

Make sure the environment is well lit. Talk with the care recipient about installing nightlights in the bedroom, bathroom, kitchen, and hallways.

Electrical cords should not be tucked under rugs or carpet.

Assist the care recipient with setting a schedule that monitors proper functioning of smoke alarms and fire extinguishers.

If appropriate, know where the care recipient keeps extra sets of household and other keys; if he or she does not want the care provider to have this information, make sure the care recipient knows where extra keys are kept.

Check water temperature at the faucets to make sure it is not too hot; have a professional or someone with experience adjust settings as needed.

Learn how to turn off gas, water, and electricity.

Emergencies

At some time or another, a care provider will be faced with an emergency situation and should be prepared to seek medical attention for the care recipient from a physician or by calling an emergency squad. Emergency phone numbers should be readily available: Write them in large print and place by each telephone. The following are suggested guidelines for knowing when to contact immediate help:

Behavior

When to call 911

Extreme lethargy
Inability to physically move or respond to physical touch
A sudden change in the ability to understand or speak clearly
Unresponsiveness or unconsciousness

When to call the doctor

Increased confusion
Hallucinations and anxiety
Change in mood or depression
Out-of-the-ordinary tiredness or lethargy
Increased agitation or aggression
Decline in functioning over several visits

Breathing

When to call 911

No breathing or breathing is difficult
Chest pain and rapid pulse
Clutching of the chest

When to call the doctor

Painful breathing
Shortness of breath
Unusual cough

Diet and Food Related

When to call 911

Choking
Ingestion of toxic chemicals or materials

When to call the doctor

Frequent, extreme thirst
Frequent lack of thirst
Loss of appetite
Significant weight loss
Difficulty chewing or swallowing food
Stomach pain before or after eating

Medications

When to call 911

Overdose
Physical consequences of taking incorrect medication

When to call the doctor

Wrong medication taken
Too much or too few of medication taken

Mobility

When to call 911

After a fall when client is experiencing pain and is unable to move with
    ease
A sudden inability to move, not as the result of a fall

When to call the doctor

After a fall, even if the care recipient does not experience pain
Persistent leg pain when walking
A change in ability to move, resulting in limited movement
Discoloration of skin in areas where there is pain
Unusual position of arms or legs
Swelling in the arms or legs
Twitching or involuntary movement

Physical

When to call 911

Numbness or tingling in hands, feet, arms, or legs combined with headache
    and dizziness
Complaints of feeling ill, with uncommon or extreme symptoms

Chest pain, pressure, or clutching of the chest
Severe bleeding
Vomiting blood
Has had a seizure lasting longer than 5 minutes
One side of the face is drooping, as a sudden change
Paralysis in an arm or leg
Severe pain in the abdomen that does not go away

When to call the doctor

Dizziness
Vomiting
Bleeding
Bedsores
Skin rashes
Excessive bruising
Unexplained swelling or redness of skin (arms, leg, face)
Discharge from wounds, sores, or other source
Frequent bladder infections

Calling 911 should not be used as a substitute for visits to the doctor or emergency room.

After repetitive calls to 911 (in some cities, even as few as three calls per person), a care recipient may be charged for emergency squad services and not all insurance policies cover these costs. Use the service when there is truly an emergency and call the physician in less urgent situations.

Telephone Contact

Cell phones and cordless phones are very handy for home care clients. A care recipient should carry these phones at all times in a purse or bag hanging from a wheelchair or walker, or strategically placed next to the bed, couch, and kitchen table. Easy access to the telephone can be essential if a care recipient falls or is unable to stand up. Tape a small piece of paper with important and emergency phone numbers to the back of the handheld telephone. Additionally, create a short cheat sheet of how to operate the telephone and put it in an easy-to-reach place.

There are unique safety measures to consider for care recipients who are confused, with Alzheimer's disease or another type of dementia, and who are not living in a supervised setting. Before making any changes to the home, discuss safety issues and concerns with the care recipient and involved family members. Together, brainstorm ideas that will maintain or increase the care recipient's safety. Special considerations and home adaptations for this type of care recipient may be to:

Disconnect the oven and stove; if the care recipient is still preparing meals, promote microwave cooking.
Remove sharp objects such as knives and other appliances that are potentially dangerous.

10.1

Exhibit

Sample emergency contact list.

Name (of client): _____

Address: _____

Phone number: _____

Family:

(Daughter) _____

(Son) _____

Emergency Contacts: <u>DIAL 911</u>

Police: 911 or _____

Ambulance: 911 or _____

Fire: 911 or _____

Doctor: 911 or _____

Nurse: _____

Neighbors:

_____   _____

_____   _____

Store cleaning supplies and toxic substances in out-of-the-way places.

Suggest the use of pillboxes that make only daily or weekly medicines available. Keep larger supplies of medications out of reach or in a locked cabinet so there is no chance the care recipient can take more pills than necessary.

Post contact names and numbers by each telephone. Exhibit 10.1 is a sample phone list.

Making the home safe and preparing the care recipient for emergencies are responsibilities of the home care provider that contribute to the success of home caregiving situations. The companion who provides supervision and monitors home safety issues makes it possible for a care recipient to remain independent, although with supervision, in their desired living environment, which may postpone the need for placement in an assisted living or nursing home. This is the goal of home care.

Household Management

Home care recipients and their family members often rely on home care providers to oversee household functioning and maintenance. Care providers are not expected to repair broken pipes or furnaces though changing light bulbs and adjusting thermostats should be anticipated. Household management is tending to routine maintenance and organization that provides safety and comfort. This includes returning items to their original place or to where the care recipient will know to look. After years of keeping the flashlight in the drawer, he or she may not think to look on the kitchen counter in a time of urgent need. Care provider tasks range from taking inventory and making lists, to operating appliances, to arranging services with specific professionals. Involve the care recipient in the process of making lists to keep track of needed supplies. When planning and organizing for the household, schedule chores and errands for specific days of the week, allowing for flexibility. Balancing care recipient needs with the allotted time schedule can be challenging in some situations; if there are time demands, prioritize tasks and errands.

There is a delicate balance of power when working on household management issues with home care recipients. To the best of his or her ability, the home care recipient should participate in discussions to make decisions and the care provider should follow those instructions and preferences. Home care providers supervise household maintenance to ensure that the care recipient is safe and living in adequate conditions, but they do not have the authority to change the lifestyle of a care recipient (see Tip 10.4). Care providers should ask enough questions to complete the project to meet client wishes and needs. Many older adults have settled into preferred practices based on years of experience. It is reassuring and comforting to care recipients in overwhelming situations that familiar routines are upheld.

Tip 10.4

Environmental Considerations for Comfort

Temperature: Set the home thermostat at a temperature comfortable for the care recipient, not the care provider. In addition to regulating room temperatures, make sure there is appropriate air circulation. Fans will keep air flowing and open windows will provide fresh air. Keep blankets and sweaters accessible to the client.

Lighting: Well-lit rooms are important for reducing eye strain as well as safety. Bright lighting is not always appropriate: Some eye conditions (i.e., cataracts) can cause a sensitivity to bright lights and shadows can cause confusion or disorientation. Proper lighting makes tasks easier to accomplish. Consider any visual limitations when adjusting the lights and ask the client what is most comfortable to him or her.

Noise: Loud noises are distracting and irritating to older people, especially if there is a hearing impairment. Sounds that contribute to high noise levels are radios, televisions, telephones, appliances, vacuum cleaners, pets, and more than one person talking at a time. Traffic, heavy equipment, and outdoor noises that can be heard inside are also disturbing; control noise levels to meet the client's comfort.

Odor: Be certain that any odors, such as electric or gasoline smells, are not cause for alarm. Eliminate odors by removing the source, not by covering the smells with perfumes and air sprays. Aromatics can be used in moderation if a client is not allergic and wishes to have the room scented.

Universal Design

Universal design is a solution-oriented concept gaining in popularity. It is intended to improve everyday living for people with disabilities, though all people can benefit from the design. The Center for Universal Design at North Carolina State University defines Universal Design as "the design of products and environments to be usable by all people, to the greatest extent possible, without the need for adaptation or specialized design" (College of Design, North Carolina State University, Center for Universal Design, 2007a). The purpose of Universal Design is to create products, homes, public buildings, and communication tools that can be used by all people regardless of age, size, or ability. Universal Design helps facilitate Aging in Place—keeping care recipients in their current living situations and making necessary arrangements for support services (see also Tip 10.5).

Tip 10.5

Home Adaptations

The American Association of Retired Persons (AARP) provides informative and how-to publications (usually free) on modifying the home. Additionally, the AARP Web site identifies common features of comfort and safety through the use of Universal Design (AARP, 2007; tips are modified for the purpose of this text from the AARP Web site):

> Barrier-free, one-story living
> No-step entry: no stairs to enter the home or main rooms
> Wide doorways and hallways for easier room-to-room mobility and to facilitate moving large things (i.e., furniture, wheelchairs) in and out of the house
> Extra floor space, which allows people with walkers or wheelchairs to have more space
> Use nonslip surfaces on floors and bathtubs
> Handrails on steps
> Grab bars in bathrooms
> Thresholds (the strip of wood on the floor in a doorway) should be flush with the floor to prevent tripping and easier access for a wheelchair to move through
> Good lighting
> Lever door handles and rocker light switches, which make opening doors and turning on lights easier for people with limited arm or hand mobility or strength.

A team of experts collaborated to define the following seven principles of Universal Design to evaluate and guide the design process for user-friendly products and environments. (NCSU, 1997b.)

Principle 1: Equitable Use

The design is useful and marketable to people with diverse abilities.

Principle 2: Flexibility in Use

The design accommodates a wide range of individual preferences and abilities.

Principle 3: Simple and Intuitive Use

Use of the design is easy to understand, regardless of the user's experience, knowledge, language skills, or current concentration level.

Principle 4: Perceptible Information

The design communicates necessary information effectively to the user, regardless of ambient conditions or the user's sensory abilities.

Principle 5: Tolerance for Error

The design minimizes hazards and the adverse consequences of accidental or unintended actions.

Principle 6: Low Physical Effort

The design can be used efficiently and comfortably and with a minimum degree of fatigue.

Principle 7: Size and Space for Approach and Use

Appropriate size and space is provided for approach, reach, manipulation, and use regardless of user's body size, posture, or mobility.

Note: Copyright 1997 by North Carolina State University, The Center for Universal Design.

These guidelines are intended to assist designers with creating products and physical spaces accessible to everyone. A home may be modified as the need arises using these principles, though the intention is to create products and build homes and public spaces to fit everyone's needs. Functional use of product and space is the primary goal of Universal Design, while balancing the need for a pleasing appearance.

Home care providers should be familiar with the idea of Universal Design. The framework of Universal Design is a source for making modifications to the home for a functional and accessible environment. Major home alterations should be left to building and construction professionals. Home care providers may need to make minor home adaptations for care recipients and should learn user-friendly approaches that could keep care recipients living longer in their own homes.

Summary

The home care provider has a responsibility to oversee home safety and take precautions that minimize or eliminate risk to the care recipient. The home care provider should regularly assess and monitor the home by identifying areas of potential hazard, and should use creative problem-solving skills to find individualized solutions that work for each care recipient. It is helpful to make a first-aid kit or other prepared kits if they are not already in the home. Nurses and physical and occupational therapists can train care providers on proper application and function of medical equipment and supplies. A home care provider should be knowledgeable about home safety routines, such as how to use a fire extinguisher, as well as the care recipient's ability to manage urgent situations. The care recipient and care provider should work together to prepare action plans for how the care recipient should react in an emergency. Preparing the care recipient for emergencies encourages self-determination and self-reliance, and overall safety. If needed, put these plans in writing and keep them in a visible place, such as on the side of the refrigerator, so the care recipient can quickly find the instructions. Also, include emergency contact phone numbers where they can be easily reached by the care recipient.

Home modifications based on the principles of Universal Design helps facilitate Aging in Place, where it is more desirable for a care recipient to not have to move to another location for care provisions. Care recipients using home care and support services are in need of assistance or else they would not have arranged services. It is likely they are unable to supervise their safety as they once did and require increased safety measures and protection. Improving home-safety routines may keep the care recipient living independently longer.

Questions

How should a care provider assess the client home for safety?
Name three home hazards that put care recipients at risk.
Are there ways to prevent falls?
What is the best practice for preventing infection?
What home adaptations can be made to improve safety?
What are simple ways to adapt the home to improve safety for a confused care recipient?
How can Universal Design benefit a home care recipient who has lived in the same home for 30 years?

Summary Tips

Regularly review home emergency procedures with client.
Talk to your local fire department to learn how to operate a fire extinguisher.

Take a CPR class to keep current on practices and techniques. The local American Red Cross chapter usually offers this course or check with your agency.

Helpful Web Sites

American Red Cross: http://www.redcross.org or contact your local chapter
Centers for Disease Control and Prevention (CDC): http://www.cdc.gov
Home adaptations and modifications (Universal Design): through AARP at http://www.aarp.org/families/home_design/universaldesign/a2004-03-23-whatis_univdesign.html
Center for Universal Design at North Carolina State University: http://www.design.ncsu.edu/cud/index.htm
Poison Control: (800) 222-1222 or contact your local Poison Center

Suggested Reading

American College of Emergency Physicians. (2003). *Pocket first aid.* New York: DK Publishing. Practical first aid.

Creative Publishing International. (2003). *The accessible home: Updating your home for changing physical needs.* Minneapolis, MN: Creative Publishing International. Creating an accessible home for persons with physical challenges.

Frechette, Leon A. (1996). *Accessible housing.* New York: McGraw Hill. Ready-to-use tools and techniques for creating a barrier-free house.

Rob, Caroline, & Reynolds, Janet. (1992). *Caregiver's guide: Helping older friends and relatives with health and safety concerns.* Boston: Houghton Mifflin. How to recognize medical and practical living problems; where and how to seek help.

Sussman, Julie, & Glakas-Tenet, Stephanie. (2002). *Dare to repair: A do-it-herself guide to fixing (almost) anything in the home.* New York: HarperCollins. A beginner's guide to home repairs.

Legal Authority and Money Matters

11

In This Chapter, You Will Learn

1. A basic understanding of legal designations for health care decision making

2. End-of-life planning

3. The importance of Advance Directives

4. The difference between Medicare and Medicaid

Why This Matters

Typically, home care recipients are able to make short- and long-term decisions that affect personal and financial situations. Home care providers take for granted that a home care recipient who lives independently has good judgment and is competent with decision-making skills, though this is not always the case. There may be a medical circumstance that creates a temporary time period when the care recipient is unable to make decisions, or a continuing decline in the care recipient's conditions that prevents good decision making. Commonly found in home caregiving situations, there can be a period of transition when the care recipient is able to function enough, even with impaired cognitive or physical skills, though is not yet ready for facility placement. A care recipient may be able to make inconsequential daily decisions, such as what activity to do for the day or what he or she will eat and wear, and continue to live at home with guidance and supervision while a family member or trusted other seeks legal authorization to make major decisions regarding health or financial issues. Home care providers should be informed if a person other than the care recipient has authority because medical and financial decisions must be processed through the legal designee for permission. Not all decision-making power is taken away from the care recipient, though if a care recipient is unable to make decisions, consent from the legal designee is needed.

Decision Making and the Older Adult

Older adults are entitled to make health care decisions independently while they are considered mentally competent and able to communicate rational and clear wishes. A physician or probate court judge has the power to deem a person mentally incompetent. At that point, legal proceedings occur to designate another person as the decision maker. Care providers should be informed if there is another person who is legally responsible to make decisions for the care recipients. In most situations, the person who has the legal authority to make financial and medical decisions is the primary caregiver, who oversees the care recipient's comfort, security, and protection.

A care provider should direct issues and concerns to the responsible person in the event of urgent or serious matters. Because this person with legal authority makes significant decisions, he or she should be notified if the care recipient is taken to the emergency room or to the doctor's office for an unscheduled, urgent appointment; if significant money matters arise; and during other nonmedical crisis situations. A care provider should follow all agency policies and protocols for contacting coworkers and responsible parties under these circumstances.

Care providers do not need to seek permission from these authorized others for everyday decisions, such as what foods the care recipient can eat or what clothing outfits he or she can wear. It is a good practice to meet with a responsible person when arranging services to understand how he or she wants to be involved with care issues and matters. This initial meeting also presents the opportunity to question limitations or restrictions placed on the care recipient.

A brief explanation of decision-making legal titles is provided here. This overview is *not* meant for the home health provider's use to recommend legal advice. Clients and family members should seek legal counsel for thorough information and advice when determining what title and role is appropriate to the caregiving situations. A care provider should involve the agency nurse or social worker, who will guide the client and family members to necessary resources.

Legal Tools and Designations for Health Care Decision Making

There are a number of legal designations that are used to give one person power to make legal, financial, and medical decisions for another person. Every legal title of power is not necessary to explain in this context, just be aware that there are several authorizations available. The three most common designations are: Durable Power of Attorney, Power of Attorney, and Guardianship. According to Black's Law Dictionary, the person who creates the document is called the "principal" or "grantor," and the person to whom power is given is called the "attorney-in-fact" or "agent" (Garner, 2004, p. 1209). Important to note is that the durable power of attorney and power of attorney instruments refer to the document and person (agent) assigned. Additionally, these two designations can only be completed while a person (principal, grantor) *is able to make competent decisions.*

Durable Power of Attorney (DPOA)

A DPOA goes into effect when the principal becomes incapacitated or unable to manage personal affairs. Black's Law Dictionary says of the DPOA, "such instruments commonly allow an agent to make healthcare decisions for a patient who has become incompetent" (Garner, 2004, p. 1210). In the event that the principal is unable to direct the course of care, the DPOA's duty is to communicate the principal's health care and end of life wishes to doctors and other health care professionals. A DPOA rarely makes financial decisions that are unrelated to health care matters; this legal designation does not grant the DPOA this authority. The DPOA should be someone who is trusted to carry out the grantor's requests because the DPOA is conveying the requested course of care the principal intended and desired. The principal must be considered mentally competent to make this designation when signing the paperwork; for this reason, it is completed before a person becomes unable to make sound decisions.

Power of Attorney (POA)

According to Black's Law Dictionary, a Power of Attorney (POA) is "an instrument granting someone authority to act as agent or attorney-in-fact for the grantor" (Garner, 2004, p. 1209). It is very similar to a DPOA. Both designations give rights to the agent to make decisions when the principal is unable. A POA can make legal, financial, and medical decisions for the principal unless a DPOA, other than the POA, has been designated.

As with a DPOA, the powers of a POA are designated before a principal becomes mentally incompetent, and go into effect when the principal (grantor) becomes incapacitated. The principal must be able to make good decisions with sound judgment in order to complete the legal paperwork and proceedings. If the principal has cognitive impairment and is deemed incompetent with decision making, the designation cannot be completed and other legal authorization arrangements, such as guardianship, will need to be considered.

Many people seek either a DPOA or a POA, not both. The POA position is more common and used frequently. If both instruments are used, the ideal situation is to have the same person as the DPOA and POA. It can become complicated if one agent is in charge of health care decisions while another agent is responsible for money matters or other nonhealth-related decisions.

The principal should choose someone who is reliable and trustworthy as his or her DPOA or POA, who will act in the principal's best interests. Health care management issues and end-of-life wishes should be clearly and precisely discussed with the DPOA or the POA.

Health care professionals rely on information and guidance from a DPOA or POA when the principal is unable to express wishes and needs. Attorneys and most physicians complete the DPOA and POA paperwork. Attorneys are obligated to keep a legal copy on file, though principals *and* agents should also keep copies of the paperwork accessible. These legal papers are critical if a care recipient is hospitalized or financial matters become urgent.

Guardianship

Black's Law Dictionary defines a guardian as "one who has the legal authority and duty to care for another's person or property, especially because of the other's infancy, incapacity, or disability" (Garner, 2004, p. 725). A guardian has the legal authority to make *all* decisions for the principal, even if it is against his or her wishes. Guardianships are enacted when a person becomes incompetent and unable to make decisions and there is no DPOA or POA designation in place. A guardian may be appointed only by a probate judge when the person-in-need (principal) is considered incompetent by a physician or the legal courts. The appointment of a guardian is effective when a person is deemed incompetent and incapable of making significant decisions.

Once a guardianship case is determined by a judge, the guardianship takes effect immediately and the principal person loses the right to make independent decisions. At the risk of losing the ability to make care and end-of-life decisions independently, guardianships are not sought until the need arises. Instead, most people plan ahead with the DPOA and POA instruments, whose power begins only when the principal is unable to make competent decisions. Typically, guardianships end at the death of the principal, though termination can occur before through legal proceedings.

Advance Directives

A Living Will, Do Not Resuscitate order, Durable Power of Attorney, and Power of Attorney documents are considered Advance Directives. These legal documents are the planning tools that designate the direction of care a principal desires for end-of-life care and decision making. Advanced Directives are used to express to family and health care professionals the wanted and unwanted types of (life-sustaining) treatments in the event that the principal is unable to communicate medical decisions. They are not tools to be used in emergency or last-minute planning. Advance Directives should be completed before crisis situations, when the principal is capable of making sound decisions.

Advance Directives can be altered while the principal is alive to reflect current wishes. For instance, a principal may have planned to have a feeding tube placed if he or she becomes unable to eat. If the principal, who is still competent, decides not to have a feeding tube or other life-sustaining measures, the documents can legally change to state these wishes. In these situations, it is critical that the principal provide up-to-date versions of these documents to the DPOA, POA, physician, and family members. Attorneys are often involved in this planning process. Be aware that laws and documents vary from state to state.

Living Will

A Living Will is the legal document that defines life-sustaining measures a principal desires if he or she becomes terminally ill. Living Wills deal with feeding tubes, intravenous (IV) fluids, and other artificial means for extending life. Many people mistake a Living Will for the document that grants a person legal authority to make health care decisions if the principal becomes incapable.

Do Not Resuscitate (DNR)

A DNR is the wish *not* to have cardiopulmonary resuscitation (CPR), which occurs when the lungs or heart stop. The DNR is designed to indicate the principal's preference to withhold life-sustaining treatments at the time of a terminal illness or permanent unconsciousness. A DNR is another Advance Directive tool. A person with a DNR order should carry a copy with them at all times. Most state laws require 911 paramedics or emergency room physicians to perform CPR *except when there is a DNR document.* The principal and designated decision maker should keep the document accessible (see Tip 11.1).

Tip 11.1

Keeping Advanced Directives Accessible

The home care recipient should keep all important legal documents in an easy-to-reach place and home care providers should be informed of where the documents are kept. Home care providers and family members will need to present these documents to paramedics, doctors, or other health care professionals in the event of an emergency and they will be necessary if the care recipient is hospitalized. (A person's will, *not* living will, does not need to be available to care providers. This is private information that should be kept in a safe place.)

Keep Advance Directives (POA, DPOA, DNR, Living Will documents) in a protective pocket on the side of the refrigerator, on top of the refrigerator, on a bookshelf, in a drawer, or in another convenient location. During an emergency, a care provider should be tending to the care recipient, not searching for these documents.

Copies of all legal documents should be given to the grantors (who have the legal authority to make decisions) and an attorney, and to any doctors who provide medical care. Formal and informal caregivers who are not responsible for making health care decisions for a care recipient do not need to have personal copies, though the documents should be accessible in the home.

Provide health care professionals with the documents during emergencies and hospitalizations; in other situations, ask the health care professional if this paperwork is needed.

Keep insurance, Medicare, and Medicaid cards and numbers readily available. Suggest that these numbers are written on a separate piece of paper and kept with other legal documents or in another convenient place for accessibility in the event of an emergency.

Money Matters: Medicare and Medicaid

The U.S. Department of Health and Human Services has two assistance programs, Medicare and Medicaid, which are often confused and misunderstood. Medicare is for people over 65 years (under 65 years *only* with particular illnesses and conditions) and people of any age in kidney (Renal) failure. Medicaid is available to low-income individuals of any age who meet the U.S. government's determined standards for income eligibility.

Medicare recipients have contributed to the government insurance program throughout their lives through monies that have been automatically deducted from an individual's payroll check. There are three programs inside of Medicare: Medicare Part A, Part B, and Part D. Medicare Part A will pay for hospitalizations and skilled nursing care in a nursing home but it does not pay for long-term stays in a facility. Many people believe that Medicare covers the full costs of long-term-care facility placement but it does not. Medicare will cover 100% of skilled-nursing-care costs for a limited time and then the percentage of costs covered will decrease over time. For example, Medicare may cover 100% of costs during the first 20 days; on the 21st day, Medicare may pay only 80% of costs, and coverage may decrease again with a longer stay in a nursing home. Medicare Part A will cover the costs for a recipient receiving skilled-nursing services or physical or occupational therapies in the home.

Participants must pay a monthly premium to receive Part B coverage, which will pay for doctor services, outpatient care, and other medical supplies and services. In a long-term-care facility, there are incidental costs of some supplies on top of basic costs that Part B will cover. Medicare Part B also covers some home health care costs.

The U.S. Congress passed the Medicare Modernization Act of 2003, a Medicare prescription drug benefit program. This law created Medicare Part D, or the Prescription Drug Plan (PDP), and was implemented in 2006 (Centers for Medicare and Medicaid Services, 2007a). The plan covers costs for generic and brand-name medications.

Everyone on Medicare is eligible for prescription drug coverage through this program: Individuals choose a plan that best suits financial means and prescription drug needs. There are numerous insurance plans within the program to choose from and the plans differ based on co-payments and the types of medications covered by each plan. A Medicare recipient must be enrolled in one of the insurance plans in order to receive prescription drug coverage. This first-ever prescription drug plan managed by the U.S. government has been controversial because of the limited medication choices within each plan. Adding to the controversy, the confusing structure of the prescription drug plan contains an overwhelming amount of information and various details to consider when choosing a prescription plan.

Medicaid covers most medical care costs once a person is enrolled in the program. There are several screening tests a person must pass in order to be Medicaid eligible. Because it is administered on the state level, a state Medicaid caseworker should be contacted for more information and an eligibility assessment.

With both Medicare and Medicaid, the money is sent directly to health care providers for delivered services. Reimbursement monies do not go to the care recipient. Medicare pays for assistance with ADL, not IADL, home care for a determined period of time. Medicaid will pay for assistance with some IADL home care if care recipients are enrolled in particular state-run programs. Medicaid is managed by individual state governments and Medicare is a federally regulated program. For more information about Medicare and Medicaid benefits and eligibility, visit the Centers for Medicare and Medicaid Services Web site through the U.S. Department of Human Services at http://www.cms.hhs.gov or contact your local Area Agency on Aging.

Summary

Advance Directives are documents and legal designations defining end-of-life care decisions when a care recipient is unable to express wishes. These measures should be put in to place before a care recipient becomes unable to direct care. Advance Directives become effective when the care recipient lacks cognitive ability to make important decisions. A Durable Power of Attorney makes health care decisions when a care recipient is deemed incompetent by legal or medical professionals. A Power of Attorney manages business and financial matters; if a Durable Power of Attorney is not assigned, the Power of Attorney will be consulted for care issues. These tools can not be implemented after a care recipient is considered incompetent; in this situation, a Guardianship is required. A Guardian is responsible for making medical and financial decisions when a care recipient is unable. Living Wills and a Do Not Resuscitate (DNR) order are specific to end-of-life treatment options because they prevent artificial, life-sustaining measures.

Medicare is a medical insurance program managed by the U.S. Federal Government. It provides for people 65 and over, with a few exceptions for persons younger. There are three major components: Part A, Part B, and Part D. Medicare Part A covers hospitalizations and skilled services (including nursing and physical and occupational therapies). Medicare Part B covers secondary medical costs, such as doctor visits, medical supplies, and some home health services. The prescription drug plan, known as Medicare Part D, is the first federally funded drug benefit program that provides coverage for some prescription medications. Medicaid is a state-regulated program for low-income people of any age. After meeting specific eligibility requirements, Medicaid will pay for most medical expenses.

Questions

What is the significant difference between a POA or DPOA and a Guardian?

When should a guardianship *not* be considered?

Should every person, regardless of age, have a Do Not Resuscitate (DNR) order?

Does a Living Will ensure a person will live longer?

Medicaid is available to every person over 65. True or False?

Which Medicare program covers home health care costs?

Medicare Part D, the prescription drug plan, covers the costs of hospitalizations. True or False?

Summary Tips

Know who will be responsible for decision making if the client is or becomes unable.

Know if the home care client has a DNR order and make sure it is readily available in the home, in case of emergency.

Be familiar with service costs covered by Medicare and Medicaid, or know who to contact and how to direct the client for additional information.

Helpful Web Sites

Centers for Medicare and Medicaid Services to learn about eligibility and benefits: http://www.cms.gov

Social Security Administration about economic issues: http://www.ssa.gov

National Academy of Elder Law Attorneys has information and education for legal services to the elderly: http://www.naela.com

American Association for Retired Persons: http://www.aarp.org

Before I Die: Medical care and personal choices at http://www.pbs.org/bid

Suggested Reading

Bove, Alexander A. (2005). *Complete book of wills, estates, and trusts*. New York: Henry Holt and Company. Easy-to-understand legal advice and information for planning health care directives.

Conklin, Joan Harkins. (2002). *Medicare for the clueless: The complete guide to government health benefits*. New York: Kensington Publishing. Understanding rules and regulations of government health benefits.

Haman, Edward A. (1998). *Power of attorney handbook*. Naperville, IL: Sourcebooks. A complete guide for health care directives and planning.

Hearn, Joseph R. (2004). *If something happens to me: A workbook to help organize your financial and legal affairs*. Omaha, NE: Provisio Publishing. Comprehensive guide with step-by-step instructions to organize financial, medical, and insurance information.

Palermo, Michael. (2004). *AARP crash course in estate planning: The essential guide to wills, trusts, and your personal legacy*. New York: Sterling Publishing. Easy-to-understand guide to estate planning.

Planning for Placement

12

In This Chapter, You Will Learn

1. How a home care provider assists client and family with long-term-care planning and decision making

2. To recognize the need for long-term-care placement

3. How to locate and research alternative living situations

4. About the care provider's role after placement in a residential facility

Why This Matters

The decision to place a loved one in any type of care facility does not happen regularly throughout life for family caregivers; usually, it is a new experience. Choosing alternative living arrangements (that is, places other than a person's home) is a major decision that can be stressful and must have successful results. Care recipients and family members often ask care providers for information pertaining to available service offerings—the extensive information can be confusing and overwhelming. Typically, home care providers have worked in health care settings and can offer insight to the advantages and disadvantages of alternative living arrangements and how facilities operate. Also, home care providers may have a more intimate understanding of care recipient needs and preferences, and family members seek this perspective. Home care providers should take the time to explain the similarities and differences in facilities and services, and how each will best serve a care recipient's needs. *Remember, home care providers are making information available, not making the decision for placement.*

Facilitating Long-Term-Care Planning

It is unlikely that a home care provider will ever need to make living arrangements or long-term-care decisions for a care recipient. Many times though, family members and professionals consult the care provider to learn of the care recipient's daily routines, habits, and preferences, which could determine the next stage of decision making. Family members and other professionals may also seek input from the care provider about the care recipient's areas of difficulty to know from the beginning what issues will need to be addressed before placement. Because a care provider tends to spend more direct, one-on-one time with the care recipient, the care provider will have insight that is helpful when planning for extended-care placement.

Moving From Home

The decision to move out of the home can be an emotional undertaking for the care recipient and family members, and it can be just as difficult to move from assisted living—even after a short time—to a long-term-care facility. Each step into a different living situation where more care is provided means to the care recipient that more assistance is necessary. A move into an assisted living or nursing home, or other supportive environment, often reveals that the care recipient is experiencing a decline and that he or she is no longer functioning independently. It is often difficult for the care recipient to admit the need for increased assistance, as it can be just as difficult for family members to recognize that there is a need for assistance. Family members—spouses and children—often feel guilty that they are not doing enough to support the care recipient in the home. A husband or wife may feel that he or she is not living up to the wedding vows of caring for the other "in sickness and in health." Children tend to view facility placement as abandoning the parent(s) who cared for them as a child, and believe that another caregiver will not be able to give the same quality of care that family provides. Other family members and even friends may have expectations of the loved one remaining in the home and may disapprove of the decision for placement.

Following are a few reasons why a care recipient may need to move out of the current living situation:

The care recipient is not able to meet personal (mental or physical) needs
The care recipient is not safe
Family members are not able to provide the level of care and assistance needed, in ongoing or crises situations
The care recipient needs more services, care, and supervision than is being provided in the home
Cost effectiveness

There are reasons for a care recipient to remain in the home and there are reasons to move into a facility. In many situations, there is no right time to move. Advantages of facility placement are considered in Table 12.1. A care recipient may choose to move because he or she realizes that the current situation is no longer manageable while other times, family members insist that the care recipient move into a supervised living situation to receive additional levels of care.

Just as there are advantages, there are also disadvantages to each alternative. See Table 12.2 for potential disadvantages. A care provider should encourage the care recipient or family members to make pro and con lists of each living alternative, specific to the wants and needs of the care recipient.

Most care recipients and families delay the discussion about facility placement. It is not a pleasant conversation. The reality is that everyone needs to think about and prepare for long-term-care arrangements, particularly if a care recipient is already receiving in-home care. The care recipient and family need to contemplate what could happen next, or should happen next, when home health care is no longer meeting care needs.

A care provider may be asked to assist the care recipient or family in gathering information about additional home care or facility services. The care provider can contribute basic advice: Plan ahead. There will be emergency events that prevent planning in some situations; for others, gathering information and preparing a general or detailed plan of action is practical, helpful, and can be crucial. For all involved with a caregiving situation, it is better to have the care recipient's wishes and wants determined ahead of time because challenging decisions should not need to be made at the last minute, during emotionally difficult times.

The care provider may act as a sounding board and offer support as the care recipient and others involved weigh factors and make decisions for alternative

12.1 Advantages of Living at Home and in a Residential Facility

Advantages of staying in the home	Advantages of moving to residential facility
• Familiar surroundings	• 24-hour supervision
• Family member will not move	• Recreational opportunities
• Cost effective	• Socialization and stimulation
• Supportive services in the home to meet client care needs	• Nursing services readily accessible
• Family members won't have negative feelings attached with facility placement	• Additional caregivers to oversee care
	• Trained professionals to manage difficult behaviors or erratic schedules
	• Stress and time constraints on family
	• Cost effective

12.2 Disadvantages of Living at Home and in a Residential Facility

Disadvantages of staying in the home	Disadvantages of moving to residential facility
• Family member stress and other obligations	• Overwhelming and unfamiliar environment
• Family unable to monitor and oversee care services	• Adjustment period where family member may have mood and behavior changes
• Behavior problems of client that produce unsafe circumstances	• Provided care does not meet standards or expectations
• Costs of in-home care	• Schedule and lifestyle changes are not suitable to familiar routines and habits
• Unable to get needed home health services	• Too much stimulation or socialization
• Unreliable home care providers	

living arrangements. A care provider can be of assistance through the processes of evaluating and choosing a residential care facility by being active in collecting information and guiding the care recipient and family to local resources. The following general outline can help a care provider and family get started in locating and researching alternative living situations.

> Learn about types of residential care facilities
> Determine care recipient's wants and needs
> Locate facilities
> Contact facilities
> Visit each facility
> Evaluate the visit
> Discuss and review information with care recipient and family

These seven steps set up a framework for the care provider to follow when assisting the care recipient and family with information gathering. These subject areas will help the care provider organize the collected information and resources to assist the care recipient and family with deciding on long-term-placement.

Living Options and Alternatives

Beyond nursing homes, most people are not familiar with the living options available until it becomes a need. Basically, there are three types of living situations: independent living, assisted living, and extended-care or nursing home placement. Independent living implies that a care recipient is self-sufficient, though may require minimal help with IADLs. People live independently in their own home or apartment, a group home, or may live in an apartment or a home in a specifically designed community for older adults. Independent living communities offer accommodating services such as dining in a restaurant-like setting, transportation, housekeeping, and activities. There are no care options in these communities unless a resident privately pays for assistance from outside resources. Assisted livings are free-standing buildings or units within extended-care facilities that are designed to promote independence but offer assistance with meals, bathing, dressing, and medications. Usually, services are set up on an as-needed basis. A care recipient may move in to an assisted living not needing much assistance and will add services as needed for an additional fee. Most assisted livings package activities, laundry, housekeeping, and three meals a day into monthly rates. Personal care routines (bathing, dressing, toileting, and feeding) become the extra, for-fee services. Other than annual health department inspections, assisted living facilities are not regulated by state or national bodies of oversight at this time. This means that assisted living amenities fluctuate from building to building, city to city, and state to state. It is not required that all assisted living facilities offer the same services; what is offered at one facility does not have to be offered at another facility. Nursing homes provide the most acute level of care and assistance of the three living situations. Most nursing homes contain a skilled-nursing unit: a hospital-like setting for care recipients who require 24-hour health care monitoring and supervision. They are often used for short-term rehabilitation visits and are staffed with therapists, nurses, nurse aides, and social workers; activity, housekeeping, and maintenance personnel; and marketing and other administrative professionals. State departments of health mandate a code of rules and regulations that apply to all nursing home facilities. These departments complete annual surveys to ensure that quality care is being provided.

Continuing Care Retirement Communities (CCRC) are campuses that offer the three aforementioned levels of care in living units across the community. On-campus living choices include private homes, independent living homes or apartments, assisted living apartments, and skilled-nursing facilities or units. The idea is that a care recipient will move into the community in independent or assisted living and as health conditions and care needs change, the care recipient will move to another living unit on the campus that provides the appropriate level of care. This arrangement is advantageous because there is an assumed continuity of care. CCRCs provide housing that meets the variety of health care needs. They also offer security: When a care recipient moves into a CCRC, he or she does not have to think about where the next level of care will come from should the need arise.

Group homes are another suitable option, though they are not in every town or city. A group home is usually a residential house where residents rent bedrooms and share common space, such as kitchen, dining, and living room areas. To learn if group homes are in your area, contact the state department of health or aging.

Determining Wants and Needs

Once the determination is made of which living situation best meets care recipient needs, the care provider, care recipient, and family members should establish criteria of what is wanted and needed from a facility. Does geographical location make a difference? Should the facility be located near family, or is it more important to choose a facility in the area that the care recipient is more familiar? Does a care recipient have a dog, which requires a facility that allows pets? Is there a need for a memory-impaired, locked unit? What type of assistance with personal care routines does the care recipient require? The cost to live in the facility and additional monthly expenses also factor into the decision.

Locating Facilities

The best way to learn about facilities is to talk with other people—friends, neighbors, acquaintances, and other health care providers. However, everyone has different experiences: What may be a successful stay for one care recipient may not have the same advantages for the next care recipient. Any residential living or care facility is only as good as the staffs who work in the facility; therefore, it is subject to change. There are other ways to learn about facilities.

- If choosing a facility that is close to family is important, drive around the community to find nearby facilities.
- Look in the yellow pages under Alzheimer's care, assisted living, nursing homes, skilled-nursing facility, retirement living, retirement and life-care communities and homes, rehabilitation, and residential care facilities. Use these as search terms on the Internet to locate services.
- Contact the local Chamber of Commerce to ask about businesses in the area.
- Call the local Area Agency on Aging or department of health.

Once facilities have been located, the next step is to contact each facility by making telephone calls and personal visits to determine which facility best provides the needed level of care and services within the care recipient's budget.

Contacting Facilities

At this point, there should be a list of what is wanted and needed from a facility and another list of potential places. Now begins the process of narrowing down the facility search. Call each residential care facility to ask fundamental questions. The responses from a facility may determine whether or not you need to make a visit. When talking to the facility representative, explain the current living situation and health conditions that are prompting the need for placement. Some questions to consider asking are:

- Can the facility manage the unique needs of the care recipient? (discuss specific needs)
- Does the facility accept care recipients with problem behaviors? (if relevant)
- Is staff trained to deal with problem behaviors? (if relevant)

What is monthly room rate?

Are there additional monthly expenses?

Is there a cost increase when a resident needs more care or supervision?

Do they accept long-term-care insurance? Medicare? Medicaid?

If the answers are satisfactory, schedule a time to meet with the facility representative for a tour, and plan on it taking at least an hour. Again, the care provider will not be making the final decision. Be sure to relay accurate information to the care recipient; as appropriate, take the care recipient and family to the facility.

Visiting and Evaluating Health Care Facilities

The world of residential care facilities has numerous options. It is an overwhelming new experience for the care recipient and family. It is more effective if the care recipient and family members tour each facility with the care provider, though sometimes the care provider will be asked to make the visit alone because family members trust the care provider's experience and knowledge. Time constraints may be an issue; family members who live out of town may not be able to quickly collect thorough information. If the care recipient is physically or cognitively unable to comprehend the planning process, the care provider may need to tour the facility alone and relay accurate information to the family. Before the tour, discuss specific questions, requests, and needs with the care recipient and family; during the tour, obtain the answers from the facility representative. Remember on each visit that this could be the care recipient's new home. Can you picture the care recipient walking comfortably into and out of this facility every day? Can you picture the care recipient's family members walking comfortably into and out of this facility for visits? Care recipients who do not have family members or significant others may need to rely on care providers, including social workers, nurses, and companions to help with long-term planning. The following general questions are for any care provider who is assisting with long-term placement and may be suggested to care recipients and family members to facilitate the placement process.

Financial Issues

Are Medicare, Medicaid, and long-term-care insurance accepted?

What types of rooms (i.e., private, suites) are available?

What is the monthly room rate for each option?

Can a resident move in to one room and be moved at a later time?

What are other unanticipated costs?

What is/is not included in the monthly rate?

What type of paperwork is needed for admission?

Resident Issues

Is there a written bill of resident rights?

Does the facility admit care recipients with Alzheimer's disease and dementia?

Is there an Alzheimer's/dementia or locked unit?
What is the process for admission?
When are mealtimes?
Can a resident be served at a different time?
Does the facility accommodate specific meal requirements and requests?
Can residents bring personal items, such as furniture and pictures?

Staffing Issues

What are the morning, day, and night staff-to-resident ratios? (One staff to how many residents?)
Is there nursing supervision 24 hours a day?
Is there a medical director available 24 hours a day?
Does staff feed residents if there is a need?
Is staff trained to manage dementia and problem behaviors?
What personal care routines will the staff assist with or provide?

Medical Issues

Can the care recipient's physician continue to treat him or her at this facility?
What hospital is used in an emergency?
What medical treatments cannot be offered at the facility?
Are Advance Directives required before admission?
Will family be contacted if there are changes in medical treatments or medications?

Therapy/Rehabilitation

Are physical, occupational, and speech therapies available in the facility?
Are there conditions of receiving therapy?
How often can the care recipient receive therapies?

Activities

Is there a weekly or monthly activity calendar?
Are group, individual, and 1:1 activities provided?
Are activities offered in evenings and on weekends?
Are there recreational outings?
Is there a family support group?

Facility Issues

Who does laundry?
How often is the room cleaned?
Are banking services available within the facility?
Are transportation services to the doctor's office or pharmacy available?
Is there a visitor policy, including visiting times?
Are doors locked at night? Is the facility secure and protected?
What is the grievance procedure, or what is the process for filing a complaint?

What is the discharge process from the facility?

Can the facility ask the resident to move out?

Ask to see results from the last annual survey completed by the State Health Department.

Stay focused on what the facility representative is saying; other questions may be more appropriate in the moment. Again, a care recipient or family may have specific questions not listed here.

In addition to asking questions, making observations during the facility tour is important. Keep in mind that accidents do happen and you may be in a facility during a crisis. On one occasion when touring an assisted living facility, the water pipes had just burst; the floors were flooded and cleaning equipment was everywhere. This is not a typical situation; rather than focusing on the problem details, observe how the staff and management deal with the disaster.

Robert, a nursing home resident, had eaten two hot dogs and macaroni and cheese with a glass of milk every day for 50 years. When he moved into a nursing home, Robert insisted on this same meal at every dinner and the facility met his demand. Nonfamily members questioned why the facility would regularly offer the unhealthy option and unbalanced diet. The nursing home allowed Robert to maintain his right to have a choice in making daily decisions. The facility's willingness to accommodate Robert's request demonstrated resident-oriented measures of individualized care. When observing other residents, be aware that many facilities do try to personalize care routines to meet individual needs. Another example is a resident who prefers to stay in bedclothes; the facility staff should accommodate this request and not insist that he or she get dressed. A resident may prefer to stay in bed late or eat meals in his or her room instead of the dining room. Some residents regularly refuse showers; they may be unclean but it is by their choice. There can be reasons that resident care looks incomplete; consider if the observations could be at a resident's request or if staff is ignoring care routines. Use good judgment: A mismatched outfit could be the resident's selection while pieces of food and stains on the clothes reflect the staff's practices.

It is important to make observations that are specific to your care recipient in addition to general observations when touring a facility:

Do most residents look clean and cared for?

Are they dressed appropriately? (i.e., is a shoe or slipper on each foot?)

Do they appear happy and content?

Are residents able to move freely around the facility?

Are your care recipient's needs consistent with the needs of the other residents?

Is your care recipient on the same functioning level of the other residents?

Will the care recipient be able to sit with residents of similar abilities?

Are the activities appropriate for varying functional levels?

Is there a variety of activity programming to meet varying needs and interests?

Are residents engaged in the activities?

Are there private visiting areas?
Is the mood in the dining room pleasant?
Are there odors?
Is the facility clean?
Are resident rooms clean?
Is the facility comfortable? Is it calm or noisy?
Is lighting adequate?
Are floor staff and management accessible?
Is staff friendly?
Is the facility in a safe neighborhood?
Is there an emergency response system facility wide? Are there pull cords
    in bathrooms?
Are resident bathrooms and shower rooms accessible?

It may be helpful to write notes as you walk with the facility representative so as not to forget the details. The care provider will need to relay details
to the care recipient and family if they are not present on the tour, and must
be conscientious to collect complete, thorough information. If questions were
not answered with a satisfaction or the care recipient and family has additional
questions, call the facility representative. The care provider may also consider
scheduling another tour to take the care recipient or a family member.

Case Study

As a companion, Judy was asked to tour an adult day care, assisted-living facilities, and nursing homes with care recipients and family members. Judy's
work experiences in various facilities made it possible for her to compare
environments and service provisions. Her understanding and knowledge of
clients' personal likes, dislikes, and preferences made it possible to identify
what would and would not work for individual clients in each setting.

Ann, a client's daughter, asked Judy to call a specific adult day care
center to get information about their service offerings. The marketing director gave Judy the necessary details. She scheduled a tour of the center
and encouraged Ann to join her. Before they even entered, they agreed
that Barbara, the care recipient, would not like the long van ride to the
center, which would mean that she would have to get up 2 hours earlier
than usual. Ann and Judy had a strong feeling that Barbara would regularly miss the transportation service. Once inside, they saw a room full of
participants but little room to move around. This limited space posed a
mobility problem for Barbara, who was overweight and used a walker. Judy
and Ann also considered that Barbara was an introvert. They thought the
large number of other attendees would be overwhelming and that Barbara
would be uncomfortable with the overstimulation. After touring and observing the center, Ann and Judy realized that this particular atmosphere
and ambiance did not fit Barbara's needs.

There are good reasons to take the care recipient on facility tours—most importantly, because it involves the care recipient in the decision-making process. This participation helps the care recipient feel that his or her opinions matter, encouraging self-determination and a sense of independence. If the care recipient attends the tour with the care provider, watch facial expressions and body language for reactions. Does the care recipient appear impressed with the surroundings? Are the activities of interest to him or her? What did he or she think about the dining room and meal presentation (if the tour occurred during a mealtime)? When interacting with staff and residents, did the care recipient seem pleased, relieved, scared, or sad?

The care recipient may experience negative emotions and reactions during or after the site visit. If it appears to be too emotionally difficult for the care recipient, keep the visit short. It is normal for a care recipient to express feelings of depression and a lack of independence, or show signs of increased agitation, forgetfulness, and suspicion. It may not be until after the tour that he or she recognizes or admits that there is need for further assistance. Regardless of how the care recipient responds to the visit, it is the care provider's responsibility to effectively listen and offer support. This is a potentially life-altering decision and it should be handled with care and consideration.

When it has been decided that the care recipient will move into an assisted living, nursing home, or continuing care retirement community, the care provider can offer suggestions that may make the move and adjustment process more successful.

Have one person—hopefully someone familiar—remain with the care recipient during the entire move-in process.

Expect the move to take several hours; avoid scheduling important appointments on the same day. The actual move might not take that long, but the care recipient may need extra time for support and reassurance.

Consider what personal possessions (i.e., furniture, pictures) should be taken to the facility.

Personalize the room with favorite and familiar objects.

Place a clock and calendar in the room. A new living environment can be confusing and overwhelming and these will help orient the new resident to day and time. It also eliminates the need for the care recipient to ask staff for that information, and until staff learns about the care recipient, these questions could be mistaken for confusion. A calendar is also a good way to keep track of visitors, appointments, and activities.

Introduce the care recipient to staff and other residents on move-in day. Do not expect that the care recipient will remember staff or resident names; it is an act to comfort the new resident and start the process of becoming familiar.

Show the care recipient around the facility; this will help to orient him or her to the new surroundings so that he or she does not have to learn the building alone or rely on staff for guidance. Do not expect that the care recipient will remember where particular rooms are located; it is an act of orientation to start the adjustment process.

Encourage the care recipient and family to decide how they will refer to the new living environment. Is it an apartment? Room? Facility? Home?

Encourage the family to visit or call frequently during the first week or more of placement. This will help the care recipient not feel as if they have been "dumped."

Encourage the care recipient or family to address concerns immediately with appropriate staff; depending on the issue, discuss issues with the marketing or admissions director, social worker, or director of nursing.

The Companion's Role After Facility Placement

A companion may or may not continue to visit and be involved with the care recipient once he or she is placed in a long-term-care facility. If the companion maintains contact with the care recipient after care facility placement, there are supportive measures with the adjustment process that the companion can offer.

The companion should introduce him- or herself to staff members. Let staff know your role and relationship with the care recipient and how often you will be visiting. The companion's role is to oversee that care routines are indeed performed and provide one-on-one attention to the care recipient. To work toward good resident care, it is important that the companion builds relationships with the staff. The more the companion is at the facility, the more comfortable staff will become with a companion's presence. The staff will need time to learn about the care recipient and should be provided with information, such as past and current likes, dislikes, habits, and preferences. Inform staff members if the care recipient has unique:

Food preferences. Not only likes and dislikes, but particular ways the care recipient prefers food to be prepared. Does he or she like ketchup on eggs? Sugar in coffee or tea? Cereal without milk? A particular menu at certain meals? Keep in mind that tastes do change.

Wake-up and bedtime routines. Does the client have habitual wake up and bed times? Are afternoon naps a must? Is the client accustomed to falling asleep with lights on or off, with the television on or music playing? Is the client particular about bedclothes? Mary had always slept in the nude. When she moved into an assisted living facility, this piece of information was not relayed to the staff. The first night Mary walked out of her room naked, staff members were startled! It was just a habit Mary had for years, nonetheless, staff considered her more confused than she actually was because of this behavior.

Personal hygiene. Is the client particular about hairstyles? How often should the client see the barber or beautician? Does the client wear nail polish? Perfume or cologne? Is style and dress important to the client?

Recreational and leisure pursuits. Is there a hobby that the client is still able to perform? Does the client like to watch television, listen to music, or have a quiet environment? Has the client ever enjoyed exercise? Are outings relaxing or overwhelming for the client? Are there particular places of interest to the client? Most families rely on the companion to monitor care at the facility and report issues and concerns back to them.

Pick your battles: Complaining about every detail is not effective and could impact the ongoing relationships with staff members. Clothes will get lost; glasses, dentures, and hearing aids will be misplaced. Direct care staff are usually helpful with these issues. Concerns with personal care routines, such as shower and toileting schedules, are best directed to supervisors. It is more productive to know to which staff and department to direct complaints. Each facility is different, so the care provider must learn about the facility's complaint procedures.

If the schedule is flexible, try visiting at various times of the day to observe what is happening with the care recipient on each shift. Are there new routines and is the care recipient adjusting? Could new care routines occur on another shift that would be easier for the care recipient? Is therapy taking place early in the morning when the care recipient is in the pattern of sleeping in? Could therapy occur in the afternoon? Also pay attention to changes in the care recipient's character and mood during the shifts. Is there a noticeable difference in demeanor from morning to night? Are particular behaviors occurring at the same time every day? Changes in routines and lifestyle are unavoidable and should be expected with residential facility placement. The companion's one-on-one attention and advocacy can aid the care recipient toward a less overwhelming transition.

Summary

The process of making decisions for home care services and residential placement can be confusing and overwhelming. There are plenty of options available, though it takes time and patience to research the services that best meet client wants and needs. Home health agencies bring services directly into the care recipient's home to encourage independent living for as long as possible. The choices of residential care settings are: independent living, group homes, assisted living, nursing homes, and continuing care retirement communities. Residential and extended-care facilities should be studied; visiting each facility, asking questions, and observing practices is the best method for choosing a new living environment. The care recipient and family will make the final decision regarding care needs and services. Care providers should offer information and resources that will assist the care recipient and family with long-term-care decision making.

Questions

When is it advantageous for a client to move out of the home and into an alternative living environment?

Identify the three levels of care and living situations.

Why is it important to involve the care recipient in decision making when planning for long-term-care placement?

Summary Tips

When touring assisted living or long-term-care facilities, take a notebook to record information, contact names and telephone numbers, questions, answers, and observations. This keeps information organized for accuracy when relaying to the care recipient or family.

Consult with a professional, such as a nurse or social worker, for long-term-placement planning.

Involve the care recipient with long-term-placement planning as much as possible. This encourages the care recipient to be active in decision making as best they are able. It may also prevent potential problems by leaving no chance for the care recipient to be surprised. In the long run, it can help make the move and transition into facility living smoother.

Helpful Web Sites

Alzheimer's Association: The Association has a program called CareFinder to help locate and choose home and residential care providers at http://www.alz.org

Assisted Living Federation of America: Advocates for quality care and accessibility for those seeking assistance with long term care at http://www.alfa.org

Eldercare Locator: Provides information for locating services in your area at 800-677-1116

Senior Housing Net: Provides resources on types of senior housing and other care services at http://www.seniorhousing.net

Suggested Reading

Baker, Beth. (2007). *Old age in a new age: The promise of transformative nursing homes*. Nashville, TN: Vanderbilt University Press. A personal journey into more than two dozen nursing homes considered the best places in America for elders to live.

Henry, Stella Mora, & Convery, Ann. (2006). *The eldercare handbook: Difficult choices, compassionate solutions*. New York: HarperCollins. A comprehensive guide to logistics and emotions of making care decisions.

Kolb, Patricia. (2003). *Caring for our elders: Multicultural experiences with nursing home placement*. Irvington, NY: Columbia University Press. Research studies on racial and ethnic influences in nursing-home placement.

References

Administration on Aging, U.S. Department of Health and Human Services. (2006). *A statistical profile of older Americans aged 65 +*. Retrieved October 27, 2007, from http://www.aoa.gov/press/fact/pdf/ss_stat_profile.pdf

Administration on Aging, U.S. Department of Health and Human Services. (2007). *Statistics*. Retrieved August 20, 2007, from http://www.aoa.gov/prof/statistics/future_growth/aging21/preface.asp

Alzheimer's Association. (2007a). *Stages of Alzheimer's disease*. Retrieved May 28, 2007, from http://www.alz.org/alzheimers_disease_stages_of_alzheimers.asp

Alzheimer's Association. (2007b). *Symptoms of Alzheimer's*. Retrieved May 28, 2007, from http://www.alz.org/alzheimers_disease_symptoms_of_alzheimers.asp

American Association of Retired Persons (AARP). (2007). *Understanding universal design*. Retrieved August 12, 2007, from http://www.aarp.org/families/home_design/universaldesign/a2004-03-23-whatis_univdesign.html

American Heart Association. (2004a). *About high blood pressure*. Retrieved May 13, 2007, from http://www.americanheart.org/presenter.jhtml?identifier=468

American Heart Association. (2004b). *Heart attack*. Retrieved May 13, 2007, from http://www.americanheart.org/presenter.jhtml?identifier=1200005

American Heritage Dictionary. (2005). *Emotional intelligence*. Retrieved May 5, 2008, from http://americanheritagedictionary.com

Arthritis Foundation. (2006). *Osteoarthritis: Understanding oa from prevention to causes and treatments*. (pp. 2–4, 10–11).

Centers for Medicare and Medicaid Services. (2007a). *Medicare program—General overview*. Retrieved June 17, 2007, from http://www.cms.hhs.gov/Medicare GenInfo

Centers for Medicare and Medicaid Services. (2007b). *Hospice payment system*. Retrieved October 13, 2007, from http://www.cms.hhs.gov/MLNProducts/downloads/hospice_pay_sys_fs.pdf

Cherniss, C. (2000). *Emotional intelligence: What it is and why it matters*. Paper presented at the Annual Meeting of the Society for Industrial and Organizational Psychology, New Orleans, LA. Retrieved July 8, 2007, from http://www.eiconsortium.org/research/what_is_emotional_intelligence.htm

College of Design, North Carolina State University, Center for Universal Design. (1997a). *About universal design, version 2.0*. Retrieved August 12, 2007, from http://www.design.ncsu.edu/cud/about_ud/about_ud.htm

College of Design, North Carolina State University, Center for Universal Design. (1997b). *The principles of universal design, version 2.0*. Retrieved August 12, 2007, from http://www.design.ncsu.edu/cud/about_ud/udprinciplestext.htm

Eden Alternative. (2007a). *Embracing elderhood*. Retrieved November 22, 2007, from http://www.edenalt.org/eden-at-home/3.html

Eden Alternative. (2007b). *Our ten principles*. Retrieved November 22, 2007, from http://www.edenalt.org/about/our-10-principles.html

Eden Alternative. (2007c). *Welcome to Eden*. Retrieved November 22, 2007, from http://edenalt.org

Eden Alternative. (2007d). *What is Eden at home*. Retrieved November 22, 2007, from http://www.edenalt.org/eden-at-home/index.html

Family Caregiver Alliance. (n.d.-a). *Selected long-term care statistics*. Retrieved March 11, 2007, from http://www.caregiver.org/caregiver/jsp/content_node.jsp?nodeid=440

Family Caregiver Alliance. (n.d.-b). *Women and caregiving: Facts and figures*. Retrieved March 11, 2007, from http://www.caregiver.org/caregiver/jsp/content_node.jsp?nodeid=892

Gall, T. (Ed.). (1998). *Worldmark encyclopedia of cultures and daily life* (vol. 3, pp. 256, 332, 466). Cleveland, OH: Eastward Publications.

Garner, B. (Ed.). (2004). *Blacks law dictionary* (8th ed.). St Paul, MN: West Publishing Company.

Klein, Gary. (2003). *Intuition at work*. New York: Doubleday.

Merriam-Webster Incorporated. (2007–2008). *Caregiver*. Retrieved March 9, 2008, from http://www.merriam-webster.com/dictionary/caregiver

Merriam-Webster Incorporated. (2007–2008). *Caretaker*. Retrieved March 9, 2008, from http://www.merriam-webster.com/dictionary/caretaker

Metropolitan Life Insurance Company Mature Market Institute. (2007). *The Metlife market survey of nursing home and health care costs*. Retrieved August 10, 2007, from http://www.metlife.com/WPSAssets/21052872211163445734V1F2006NHHCMarketSurvey.pdf

National Cancer Institute. (2007). *Cancer: Questions and answers*. Retrieved June 1, 2007, from http://www.cancer.gov/cancertopics/factsheet/Sites-Types/general

National Institute of Mental Health. (2007). *NIH senior health: Depression*. Retrieved October 26, 2007, from http://nihseniorhealth.gov/depression/faq/faq2a.html

National Institute of Neurological Disorders and Stroke. (2007). *Parkinson's disease: Hope through research*. Retrieved June 3, 2007, from http://www.ninds.nih.gov/disorders/parkinsons_disease/detail_parkinsons_Disease.htm#90573159

The President's Council on Bioethics. (2002). *The promise and the challenge of aging research*. Retrieved April 29, 2007, from http://www.bioethics.gov/background/agingresearch.html

Russell, C. (2000). *Demographics of the U.S.: Trends and projections*. Ithaca, NY: New Strategist Publications.

U.S. Bureau of Labor Statistics. (2007). Retrieved March 11, 2007, from http://www.stats.bls.gov/opub/mlr/2007/11/art4full.pdf

U.S. Census Bureau. (2004). *Projected population of the United States by age and sex: 2000–2050* (Table 2a). Retrieved October 27, 2007, from http://www.census.gov/ipc/www/usinterimproj/natprojtab02a.pdf

U.S. Department of Agriculture. (2007). *Dietary guidelines 2005*. Retrieved September 15, 2007, from http://www.health.gov/dietaryguidelines/dga2005/document/html/chapter2.htm#table1

Index

Abbreviations, for health care, 38–39
Activities, 131–161
  action plan example, 134
  active and passive participation,
    134–135
  activities of life and activities of
    recreation, 135–137
  art galleries and gift shops, 153
  case study, 141
  chair exercises, 145–146
  companion's role in activity planning,
    137–139
  cooking and baking, 143
  enjoying the outdoors from inside, 151
  food as fun, 152–153
  gardening, 142–143
  garden stores and nurseries, 152
  golf, 145
  greenhouses and gardens
    (conservatories), 151–152
  for impaired persons, 157–158
  in long-term-care facilities, 230
  magazine treasure hunt, 147
  mind mapping, 146–147, 157, 159
  museums, 153–154
  music, 148–150
  outdoor stimulation, 144
  parks, 151
  preparing for, 139–140
  puzzles and board games, 148
  quality of life and, 132–135
  quilt stores, 153
  reminiscing, 154–157
  shopping, 142
  tips for choosing, 140
  walking, 144–145
  Web sites for, 160
  word games, 147–148
Activities of Daily Living (ADLs), 32, 135
  defined, 16–17
  tasks, 17
  See also Activities; Skilled care
Activity action plan (example), 134

ADLs. See Activities of Daily Living
Administration on Aging (DHHS), 4
Adult day care, 21
Advance Directives, 217–219
  See also Legal authority
African Americans
  health care providers of, 8
  over 65 years, 4
Ageism, 2–3
Agent (attorney-in-fact), 217
Age-related changes, 5, 78–79
Age-related conditions. See Diseases
Aging
  normal, 5–8
  nutrition and, 164–169
Aging population, 22
  Baby Boomer Generation, 22–24
  statistics on, 23
Air mattress, 193
Alcoholism, 79–80
Alzheimer's disease, 13, 80–84
  seven stages of (Global Deterioration
    Scale), 81–82
  special diets and, 165
American Red Cross, 204
Anxiety disorder, 106
Appearance, 67
Art galleries, 153
Arthritis, 84–85
Asian/Pacific Islanders
  health care providers of, 8
  over 65 years, 4
Assisted living communities, 227
Attentive listening, 59–60
Attitudes
  on aging, 2–3
  on caregiving, 13–14
Attorney-in-fact (agent), 217

Baby Boomer Generation, 22–24, 12
  statistics, 23
Baking, 143
Bath bench, 196

Bathroom equipment, 195–198
Bathroom safety, 189
  equipment for, 195–198
Bed canes, 193
Bed pads, 195
Bed pans, 195
Bed rails, 193
Bedside commode, 195
Bedsores, 85–86
Bed wedges, 195
Behavior emergencies, 205
Black's Law Dictionary, definitions of
  Advance Directives, 217–219
Blanket support, 195
Bleeding, 187
Board games, 148
Boundaries, establishing, 43–44
Brace, 200
Breathing emergencies, 205
Burnout, 43–44
Burns, 187

Calcium, 168
Cancer, 86–88
Canes, 191, 193
Can opener, 198
Cards, 155
Caregivers, 12–15
  defined, 12
  types of, 12
  See also Home care providers
    (Nonmedical); Informal caregivers
Caregiving
  attitudes on, 13–14
  statistics on, 15
  Web sites for, 28–29
Case studies
  activities, 141
  couples, 127–128
  home care providers, 32–33, 34–35,
    40–41
  long-term-care placement, 232
  safety, 184–185
Cerebral vascular accident, 112–113
Chair exercises, 145–146
Cherniss, Cary, "Emotional Intelligence:
  What It Is and Why It Matters", 48
CHF. *See* Congestive heart failure
Chicken parmesan, 174
Chicken salad, 173
Chronic obstructive pulmonary disease
  (COPD), 105
Cognitive skills, 133
Communication skills, 52–74
  conflict-resolution skills, 63–65
  conversation skills, 56–58

decision-making skills, 65–66
with family, 55–56
listening skills, 58–60
observation skills, 66–74
problem-solving skills, 60–63
Web sites for, 75
See also Observation skills; Skills
Community-based services, 20
Companion care, 32–35
  duties of, 18–19
  role of after facility placement, 234–235
  salaries for, 13
  See also Home care providers
    (nonmedical)
Compassion, 52
Conflict-resolution skills, 63–65
Congestive heart failure (CHF), 88
Conservatories, 151–152
Constipation, 89–90
Continence, 90–92
Conversation skills, 56–58
Cooking, 143, 158
  safety and, 201
  See also Meals; Recipes
COPD. *See* Chronic obstructive
  pulmonary disease
Costs, 12
Couch cane, 193, 198
Counseling, 20
Couples, 125–130
  caring for, 126
  case study, 127–128
  defining couples, 128–129
  emotions of partners in care, 126–127
  respite care, 129
  situations of partner care, 126
  Web sites for, 130
Culture, different attitudes on aging, 3, 8
Curry in a hurry (recipe), 178
Cushions, 199
Cyanosis, 120

Daily acitivity log, 37
Daily life coping skills, 6–7
Day care, 21
Death rates, 22
Decision-making skills, 65–66
Dementia, 13, 92–93
Dependency, 2, 6
Depression, 93–95
  statistics on, 3
Diabetes, 95–96, 166
Diabetic diet, 165
Diet and food related emergencies, 206
Dietary guidelines, 167–169
Diets, special, 165–167

Disasters, 203–204
Discomfort, changes in, 70
Discrimination, positive and negative, 3
Diseases, 2–3, 77–115
    the aging body, 78–79
    alcoholism, 79–80
    Alzheimer's disease, 80–84
    arthritis, 84–85
    bedsores, 85–86
    cancer, 86–88
    congestive heart failure (CHF), 88
    constipation, 89–90
    continence, 90–92
    dementia, 92–93
    depression, 93–95
    diabetes, 95–96
    gastroesophageal reflux disease
        (GERD), 96–98
    hearing loss, 98–99
    heart disease, 99–100
    high blood pressure (HBP/
        hypertension), 100–102
    impaired and loss of vision, 102–103
    kidney disorder (renal disease), 103–104
    lung disease, 104–106
    mental health, 106–107
    osteoporosis, 107–108
    pain, 108–109
    Parkinson's disease, 109–111
    physicians and specialists, 113–114
    statistics, 113
    stroke (CVA/cerebral vascular
        accident), 112–113
    Web sites for, 115
Disposable gloves, 203
DNR. *See* Do Not Resuscitate
Documentation, 36–37
Do Not Resuscitate (DNR), 219
Dopamine, 109
DPOA. *See* Durable Power of Attorney
Dressing, 34
Durable Power of Attorney (DPOA), 217

Eating habits, 69–70
Economic issues, 13
Eden Alternative at home, 25–27
Egg carton pad, 193
Egg salad, 174
EI. *See* Emotional Intelligence
Elderhood, 27
Electric scooter, 192
E-mail correspondence, 36
Emergencies, 205–208
Emergency contact list, 201, 204, 208
Emergency response button, 200
Emergency supply kits, 203–204

"Emotional Intelligence: What It Is and
    Why It Matters" (Cherniss), 48
Emotional Intelligence (EI), 47–48
Emotional Intelligence (Goleman), 47
Emotions
    of caring for others, 42–44
    of partners in care, 126–127
Employment
    average hourly rate for companion care
        providers, 13
    statistics of home care providers, 21–22
End of life wishes, 217
    See also Legal authority
Environmental considerations, in the
    household, 209
European Americans
    over 65 years, 4
    view of disease, 8
Everyday tasks, 17
    See also Activities; Instrumental
        Activities of Daily Living (IADLs)
Exercising, 143–146, 158
Extended-care facilities, 227
    See also Long-term-care placement;
        Nursing homes

Facility issues, long-term-care placement
    and, 230–232
Facility placement. *See* Long-term-care
    placement
Fainting (syncope), 187–188
Falls, preventing, 189–190
Family
    communicating wih, 55–56
    See also Caregivers; Informal
        caregivers
Family Caregiver Alliance, 21–22
Fiber, 168
Financial issues, long-term-care
    placement and, 229
Finger-food diet, 165
Fire extinguishers, 201
Fireplaces, 201
Fire safety, 201
First-aid kit, 186–187
Food
    as fun, 152–153
    See also Meals; Recipes
Formal caregivers
    defined, 14
    See also Activites of Daily Living
        (ADLs)

Gait belt, 192
Games, 146–148, 158
    See also Activities

Gardening, 142–143
Gardens, 151–152
Garden stores, 152
Gastroesophageal reflux disease (GERD), 78, 96–98
GDS. *See* Global Deterioration Scale
Geographic issues, 13
GERD. *See* Gastroesophageal reflux disease
Gift shops, 153
Global Deterioration Scale (GDS) (Seven Stages of Alzheimer's disease), 81–82
    See also Alzheimer's disease
Goleman, Daniel, *Emotional Intelligence*, 47
Golf, 145
Government-sponsored programs, 3
Grab bars, 198
Grabber/reacher, 199
Grab ropes, 199
Grantor (principal), 217
Greenhouses, 151–152
Grief, stages of, 118–119
Group homes, 227
Guardianships, 218

Handheld shower, 196–197
Hand washing, 202–203
HBP. *See* High blood pressure
Hearing, 70–71
Hearing devices, 190
Hearing loss, 98–99
Heart disease, 99–100
High blood pressure (HBP/hypertension), 100–102
Hispanic Americans, health care providers of, 8
Hoehn and Yahr Scale (Parkinson's disease), 110–111
Home adaptations, 210
Home care
    choosing, 18–21
    cost of vs. nursing home care, 22
    defined, 16
    Eden Alternative, 25–27
Home care clients, rights of, 24–25
Home care industry, 21–25
Home care providers (nonmedical), 31–50
    caregiver burnout, 43–44
    case studies, 32–33, 34–35, 40–41
    companions, 32–35
    e-mail correspondence and, 36
    emotions of caring for others, 42–44
    goals and objectives of, 39–40
    health care abbreviations, 38–39
    quality traits of, 45

roles and responsibilities, 35–36
    sample daily activity log, 37
    self care of, 45–48
    Web sites for, 49
    working with others, 40
    See also Companion care; Instrumental Activities of Daily Living (IADLs)
Home-delivered meals, 19
Home health care, defined, 16
Home infusion equipment, 201
Homemakers, duties of, 18–19
Hospice care, 120–122
    See also Palliative care
Hospital bed, 193
Household activities, 68, 141–143, 157–158
Household management, 68, 208–212
    environmental considerations for comfort, 209
    home adaptations, 210
    universal design, 210–212
    Web sites for, 213
    See also Instrumental Activities of Daily Living (IADLs)
Hydraulic lift, 194
Hypertension, 100–102

IADLs. *See* Instrumental Activities of Daily Living
Impaired care recipients, activities for, 157–158
Independent living communities, 227
Infection control, 202–203
Informal caregivers, defined, 14
    See also Caregivers
Instrumental Activities of Daily Living (IADLs), 32, 135
    defined, 16–17
    tasks, 17
    See also Activities; Home care providers (nonmedical); Nonskilled care
Insurance industry, 2
Insurance policies, long-term-care, 4
Interpersonal skills. *See* Skills
Interpretation skills, 73–74
Intuition, 72
Italian tofu and spinach patties, 179

Jewish Kosher diet, 166

Kidney disorder (renal disease), 103–104
    Medicare coverage and, 220
Kitchen safety, 201–202
Klein, Gary, 77
Kubler-Ross, Elisabeth, grief stages, 118

Lazy Susan, 198
Legal authority, 216–220
    Advance Directives, 218–219
    Do Not Resuscitate (DNR), 219
    Durable Power of Attorney (DPOA), 217
    Guardianship, 218
    legal document accessiblity, 219–220
    Power of Attorney (POA), 217–218
    Web sites for, 222
Legal documents, accessiblitiy of, 219–220
Life expectancy, 12, 22
Lift chair, 198, 199
Liquid diet, 166
Listening skills, 58–60
    attentive listening, 59–60
    See also Communication skills;
        Obversation skills; Skills
Live music, 149
Living Wills, 219
Long-handled sponge, 197
Long-term-care insuance policies, 4
Long-term-care placement, 223–236
    activities offered, 230
    advantages of moving from home, 224–225
    assisted living, 227
    case study, 232
    companion's role after facility placement, 234–235
    contacting facilities, 228–229
    determining wants and needs, 227–228
    disadvantages of moving from home, 225–226
    facility issues, 230–231
    finanical issues, 229
    group homes, 227
    independent living communities, 227
    locating facilities, 228
    medical issues, 230
    move-in and adjustment process, 233–234
    nursing homes/extended-care, 227
    observations to make while touring facilities, 231–232
    resident issues, 229–230
    staffing issues, 230
    therapy/rehabilitation issues, 230
    Web sites for, 236
Low-fat diets, 166
Low-sodium diet, 165–166
Lung disease, 104–106

Magazine treasure hunt, 147
Male urinal, 195

Meals, 163–182
    assistance during, 171
    dietary guidelines, 167–169
    involving the client in planning and preparation, 169–171
    monitoring, 169
    nutrition, 164–169
    quick cooking and planning, 179–180
    recipes, 173–180
    shopping for the client, 171–173
    special diets, 165–167
    vitamins and minerals, 167–168
    Web sites for, 181
    See also Recipes
Mechanical-soft diet, 165
Medicaid, 221
    Web site for, 221, 222
Medical equipment, 19, 190–201
Medical issues, long-term-care placement and, 230
Medicare, 3
    descriptions of Parts A, B, and D, 220–221
    hospice care and, 121–122
    Web site for, 221, 222
Medicare Modernization Act (2003), 220–221
Medication emergencies, 206
Memory changes, normal, 81
    See also Alzheimer's disease;
        Dementia
Men, over 65 years, 4
Mental health disorders, 106–107
Mental incompetency, health care decisions and, 216
Metropolitan Life Insurance Company Mature Market Institute, 13
Mind mapping, 146–147, 157, 159
Minerals, 167–168
Minorities, over 65 years, 4
Mobility emergencies, 206
Money management, 20
Mood, 67–68
Motorized scooter, 192
Move-in and adjustment process, 233–234
Museums, 153–154
Music, 148–150
Myths, 3–5

NAHC. *See* National Association for Home Care & Hospice
National Association for Home Care & Hospice (NAHC), Bill of Rights for care recipients, 24–25

National Family Caregivers Association (NFCA), 12–13
National Institute of Mental Health, depression statistics, 3
National Institute of Neurological Disorders and Stroke, 109
National Institute on Alcohol Abuse and Alcoholism (NIAAA), definition of alcoholism, 79
Native Americans
health care providers of, 8
over 65 years, 4
Natural disasters, preparing for, 203–204
NFCA. *See* National Family Caregivers Association
NIAAA. *See* National Institute on Alcohol Abuse and Alcoholism
Nonmedical support services, as business, 35
See also Companion care; Home care providers (nonmedical); Instrumental Activities of Daily Living (IADLs)
Nonskilled care, 14
duties of, 16–17
See also Instrumental Activities of Daily Living (IADLs)
Normal aging, 5–8
Nurse aides, duties of, 19
Nurseries, 152
Nurses, duties of, 19
Nursing homes, 227
costs of vs. companion care, 13, 22
statistics on, 4
See also Extended-care facilities; Long-term-care placement
Nutrition, 164–169
See also Dietary guidelines; Meals; Recipes

Observation skills, 66–74
appearance, 67
changes in pain or discomfort, 70
eating and sleeping habits, 69–70
hearing, 70–71
for the household, 68
interpretation, 73–74
intuition, 72
mood, 67–68
for personal care, 68–69
seeing, 71
smelling, 71
tasting, 71–72
touching, 72
Obsessive compulsive disorder (OCD), 106
OCD. *See* Obsessive compulsive disorder
Osteoporosis, 107–108

Outdoor activities, 142–145, 150–152
See also Activities
Outdoor stimulation, 144
Outings, 152–154
Oxygen tank, 200–201

Pain, 108–109
changes in, 70
Paki-beef (recipe), 177
Palliative care, 120
See also Hospice care
Parkinson's disease, 109–111
Hoehn and Yahr scale for, 110–111
Parks, 151
Part A, of Medicare, 220
Part B, of Medicare, 220
Part D, of Medicare (prescription drug coverage), 220–221
Pasta primavera (recipe), 174–175
Patience, 52
Peanut butter noodles (recipe), 178–179
Personal care routines, 17, 68–69
See also Activities of Daily Living (ADLs)
Personal growth, 47–48
Personalizing activities, 46–47
Personal skills, 52
Pharmaceuticals, 2
Physical changes, 5
Physical emergencies, 206–207
Physical skills, 133
Physicians, 113–114
Pillows, 199
Pizza (recipe), 176–177
Placement. *See* Long-term-care placement
Plate guard, 198
POA. *See* Power of Attorney
Portable commode, 195
Posttraumatic stress disorder (PTSD), 106
Power of Attorney (POA), 217–218
Prescription Drug Plan (PDP) Part D of Medicare, 220–221
Principal (grantor), 217
Problem-solving skills, 60–63
Professional growth, 47–48
Protein, 168
PTSD. *See* Posttraumatic stress disorder
Pureed diet, 165
Puzzles, 148

Quad cane, 191
Quality of life, activities and, 132–135
Quilt stores, 153

Raised toilet seat, 197
Ramp, 199, 200
Reading, 158
Recipes, 173–180
　chicken parmesan, 174
　curry in a hurry, 178
　egg salad, 174
　Italian tofu and spinach patties, 179
　paki-beef, 177
　peanut butter noodles, 178–179
　red beans and rice, 177–178
　stuffed green pepper soup, 176
　tomato-free pizza, 176–177
　tuna or chicken salad, 173
　vegetable pasta primavera, 174–175
　vegetable soup, 175–176
Red beans and rice, 177–178
Reisberg, Barry, 81
Relaxation, 132
Religious beliefs, 7–8
Reminiscing, 154–157
Renal disease, 103–104
Residential facilities, 226–227
Resident issues, long-term-care
　placement and, 229–230
Residiential facilities. See Long-term-
　care placement
Respite care, 19, 129
Responsibilities, of home care providers,
　35–36
Rheumatoid arthritis, 84
Rights, of home care clients, 24–25
Roles and responsibilities, of home care
　providers, 35
Rubber bath mat, 197

Safety, 184–208
　bathroom safety, 189
　case study, 184–185
　fire safety, 201
　first-aid kit, 186–187
　general safety in the home, 204–205
　infection control, 202–203
　kitchen safety, 201–202
　medical equipment and supply safety,
　　190–201
　natural disasters, 203–204
　preventing falls, 189–190
　Web sites for, 213
Safety bars, 198
Salaries, of companion care providers, 13
Scooters, 192
Seeing, 71
Segregation, 3
Seizures, 188
Self care, of caregivers, 45–48

Senior centers, 20–21
Senses, observing, 70–72
Sensory perceptions, 5
Sensory skills, 133
Shopping, 142
　for the client, 171–173
　special diets and, 166–167
Shopping list, 172–173
Shower seat, 196
Singing, 150
Skilled care, duties of, 16–17
　See also Activities of Daily Living
　　(ADLs)
Skills, 51–76, 133
　communication skills, 52–58
　conflict-resolution skills, 63–65
　conversation skills, 56–58
　decision-making skills, 65–66
　listening skills, 58–60
　observation skills, 66–74
　personal skills, 52
　problem-solving skills, 60–63
　Web sites for, 75
　See also Communication skills;
　　Observation skills
Sleeping habits, 69–70
SMART, 40
Smelling, 71
Smoking, 201
Social issues, 12–13
Social skills, 133
Social stimulation, 7
Society for Industrial and Organizational
　Psychology, 48
Soups, 175–176
Special diets, 165–167
Specialists, 113–114
Spiritual beliefs, 7–8
Staffing issues, long-term-care placement
　and, 230
Stair lift, 199–200
Statistics
　on aging population, 22
　on Americans over 65 years, 4
　on Baby Boomer Generation, 23
　of caregiving, 15
　caregiving Web sites, 28–29
　on depression, 3
　of health and chronic conditions, 113
　of home care industry, 21–22
　on nursing homes, 4
Stereotypes, 3
Straight cane, 191
Stress, reducing, 45–46
Stroke (CVA/cerebral vascular accident),
　112–113

Stuffed green pepper soup (recipe), 176
Supply safety, 190–201
Swivel spoon, 198
Symptoms
  alcoholism, 79–80
  Alzheimer's disease, 82–83
  arthritis, 84
  bedsores, 85
  cancer, 86–87
  congestive heart failure (CHF), 88
  constipation, 89–90
  continence, 91
  dementia, 92–93
  depression, 94
  diabetes, 95–96
  gastroesophageal reflux disease
    (GERD), 96–98
  hearing loss, 98
  heart disease, 99–100
  high blood pressure, 101
  kidney disorder, 103
  lung disease, 105
  mental health disorders, 106
  osteoporosis, 107–108
  pain, 108
  Parkinson's disease, 110
  stroke, 112
  vision, impaired or loss of,
    102–103
Syncope (fainting), 187–188

Tasting, 71–72
Telephones, 207–208
Terminal illness, 117–123
  diagnosis and, 118
  grief stages (Kubler-Ross), 118–119
  hospice care, 120–122
  physical changes, 119–120
  Web sites for, 123
Therapy/rehabilitation in long-term-care
  facilities, 230
Thickened liquids, 165
Thomas, William, 25, 27
Tinnitus, 98
Toilets, 197
Toilet safety frame, 197
Tomato-free pizza (recipe), 176–177
Touching, 72
Touring facilities, 229–234
Transfer bench, 196
Transfer board, 192
Transportation, 20
Trapeze bar, 194
Treatment
  alcoholism, 80
  Alzheimer's disease, 83
  arthritis, 84–85

bedsores, 86
cancer, 87
congestive heart failure (CHF), 88
constipation, 90
continence, 91
dementia, 93
depression, 94
diabetes, 96
gastroesophageal reflux disease
  (GERD), 96–98
hearing loss, 98–99
heart disease, 100
high blood pressure, 101
kidney disease, 104
lung disease, 105
mental health disorders, 107
osteoporosis, 108
pain, 109
Parkinson's disease, 111
stroke, 112
vision, impaired or loss of, 102–103
Tuna salad, 173
Two-wheeled walker, 191

Universal design, 210–212
Universal Precautions, for infection
  control, 202
Urinal, 195
U.S. Department of Agriculture, dietary
  guidelines, 167
U.S. Department of Health and Human
  Services, Medicare and Medicaid, 220

Vegetable pasta primavera (recipe),
  174–175
Vegetable soup (recipe), 175–176
Vegetarians, 166
Vision, impaired or loss of, 102–103
Visual aids, 190
Vitamins, 167–168

Walkers, 191
Walking, 144–145
Web sites, 9
  activities, 160
  alcoholism, 80
  Alzheimer's disease, 84
  American Association for Retired
    Persons, 222
  arthritis, 85
  bedsores, 86
  cancer, 88
  caregiving information, education,
    trends, and statistics, 28–29
  congestive heart failure (CHF), 88
  constipation, 90
  continence, 92

couples, 130
dementia, 93
heart disease, 100
high blood pressure, 102
home care providers, 49
household management, 213
kidney disorder, 104
long-term-care placement, 236
lung disease, 106
meals, 181
Medicare and Medicaid, 221, 222
mental health disorders, 107
safety, 213
skills, 75

Social Security Administration, 222
state senators, 28
stroke, 113
the terminally ill, 123
vision, impaired or loss of, 103
Wheelchairs, 191
Women
    caregiving and, 12, 14
    over 65 years, 4
Word games, 147–148
Worldmark Encyclopedia of Cultures and Daily Life (Gall), 2–3

Young-old, 3

SPRINGER PUBLISHING COMPANY

Bathing Without a Battle

Person-Directed Care of Individuals With Dementia, Second Edition

Ann Louise Barrick, PhD; Joanne Rader, RN, MN
Beverly Hoeffer, DNSc, RN, FAAN; Philip D. Sloane, MD, MPH
Stacey Biddle, COTA/L, Editors

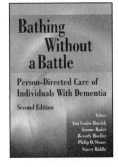

Like its popular predecessor, the new edition of *Bathing Without a Battle* presents an individualized, problem-solving approach to bathing and personal care of individuals with dementia. On the basis of extensive original research and clinical experience, the editors have developed strategies and techniques that work in both institution and home settings. Their approach is also appropriate for caregiving activities other than bathing, such as morning and evening care, and for frail elders not suffering from dementia.

For this second edition, the authors have included historical material on bathing and substantially updated the section on special concerns, including:

- Pain
- Skin care
- Determining the appropriate level of assistance
- Transfers
- The environment

An enhanced final section addresses ways to support caregivers by increasing their understanding of the care recipient's needs and their knowledge of interventions to improve care and comfort. It also emphasizes self-care and system-level changes to promote person-directed care. Several chapters include specific insights and wisdom from direct caregivers.

Partial Contents:

Part I: The Basics
- Understanding the Battle
- Temperatures of the Times: Fluctuations in Bathing Through the Ages
- General Guidelines for Bathing Persons With Dementia
- Assessing Behaviors
- Selecting Person-Directed Solutions That Work

Part II: Special Concerns
- Person-Directed Care: Sustaining Interactions Through Offering the Needed Level of Assistance
- Managing Pain
- Care of the Skin
- Transfer Techniques
- The Physical Environment of the Bathing Room
- Equipment and Supplies

Part III: Supporting Caregiving Activities
- Bathing as a Vehicle for Change
- Interactive Approaches to Teach Person-Directed Bathing
- Taking Care of Yourself: Strategies for Caregivers

March 2008 · 208 pp · Softcover · 978-0-8261-0124-2

11 West 42nd Street, New York, NY 10036-8002 • **Fax: 212-941-7842**
Order Toll-Free: 877-687-7476 • **Order Online: www.springerpub.com**

SPRINGER PUBLISHING COMPANY

Caregiving Contexts
Cultural, Familial, and Societal Implications

Maximiliane E. Szinovacz, PhD
Adam Davey, PhD, Editors

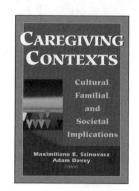

"This volume represents a major step forward in the literature by placing its focus squarely on the caregiving context, its dimensions and how it shapes the process and outcomes of family care. The chapters locate care within the family, rather than a single individual....The family, in turn, is embedded within a larger cultural, community, and social context....These explorations of context will give us a broader view of how caregiving occurs. It will help us improve our theories about care and about the family's role in contemporary society....Care of our elders is an enduring and yet evolving part of life. The focus on context will help us understand, support and learn from the ways that families meet the challenges involved."

—From the Foreword by **Steve H. Zarit,** PhD
Professor and Head, Department of Human Development and
Family Studies, Pennsylvania State University

Here in **Caregiving Contexts,** the editors and their chapter authors explore the ways in which demographic change will influence the availability of caregivers and how divergent welfare and ideological systems will affect care among family members and between family and formal care systems. They also discuss the differences in experience between spousal and adult child caregivers, special circumstances such as child or adolescent caregivers, and government and workplace policies that are available to support caregivers in the United States and in some European countries.

No other volume is available on caregiving that explores the sociocultural, familial, and sociopolitical contexts that affect both care decisions and outcomes.

2007 · 312 pp · Hardcover · 978-0-8261-0287-4

11 West 42nd Street, New York, NY 10036-8002 • Fax: 212-941-7842
Order Toll-Free: 877-687-7476 • Order Online: www.springerpub.com